I0413236

Estimated Withdrawals and Use of Water in Colorado, 2005

By Tamara Ivahnenko and Jennifer L. Flynn

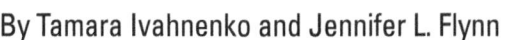

Prepared in cooperation with the Colorado Water Conservation Board

Scientific Investigations Report 2010–5002

U.S. Department of the Interior
U.S. Geological Survey

U.S. Department of the Interior
KEN SALAZAR, Secretary

U.S. Geological Survey
Marcia K. McNutt, Director

U.S. Geological Survey, Reston, Virginia: 2010

For more information on the USGS—the Federal source for science about the Earth, its natural and living resources, natural hazards, and the environment, visit http://www.usgs.gov or call 1-888-ASK-USGS

For an overview of USGS information products, including maps, imagery, and publications, visit http://www.usgs.gov/pubprod

To order this and other USGS information products, visit http://store.usgs.gov

Suggested citation:
Ivahnenko, Tamara, and Flynn, J.L., 2010, Estimated withdrawals and use of water in Colorado, 2005: U.S. Geological Survey Scientific Investigations Report 2010–5002, 61 p.

Contents

Abstract 1

Introduction 2

    Purpose and Scope 2

    Sources of Data 2

    Limitations of the Data 5

    Methods of Analysis 5

Estimated Withdrawals and Uses of Water in 2005 5

    Water Withdrawals by Category 6

        Irrigation 15

        Public Supply 18

        Self-Supplied Domestic 23

        Self-Supplied Industrial 23

        Livestock 23

        Mining 28

        Thermoelectric 31

        Instream Hydroelectric Power Generation 36

        Other Water Uses 36

    Water Withdrawals by Selected Aquifer 38

    Comparison of the Colorado Statewide Water Supply Initiative Baseline
        Forecasted Water Demand for 2005 to Select 2005 Water-Use Estimates 38

    Comparison of 1985 to 2005 Colorado Compilation Water Withdrawal Estimates 46

Summary 47

Acknowledgments 49

References Cited 49

Glossary 51

Appendix 53

Figures

1–12.   Maps showing:

        1.   Major river basins and hydrologic unit code numbers in Colorado 3

        2.   Counties and select cities in Colorado 4

        3.   Interbasin water transfers between hydrologic subregions 6

        4.   Estimated total water withdrawals by Colorado county, 2005 12

        5.   Estimated total water withdrawals by four-digit hydrologic unit codes,
            Colorado, 2005 14

        6.   Estimated total irrigation (crop and golf course) water withdrawals by
            Colorado county, 2005 19

        7.   Estimated total public-supply water withdrawals by Colorado county,
            2005 22

        8.   Estimated total self-supplied domestic-water withdrawals by Colorado
            county, 2005 26

9. Estimated total self-supplied industrial-water withdrawals by Colorado county, 2005 27
10. Estimated total mining water withdrawals by Colorado county, 2005 34
11. Locations of coal, natural gas and other fossil-fuel (water cooled), and hydroelectric power generating facilities in Colorado, 2005 35
12. Denver Basin aquifers, Colorado 39

Tables

1. Interbasin water transfers between hydrologic subregions, 2005, Colorado 7
2. Total population and water withdrawals in Colorado by county, 2005 9
3. Total population and water withdrawals in Colorado by hydrologic unit code, 2005 13
4. Estimated crop irrigation water withdrawals in Colorado by county, 2005 16
5. Estimated public-supply water withdrawals and deliveries in Colorado by county, 2005 20
6. Estimated self-supplied domestic-water withdrawals in Colorado by county, 2005 24
7. Estimated self-supplied industrial-water withdrawals in Colorado by county, 2005 28
8. Livestock water requirements 28
9. Estimated livestock water withdrawals in Colorado by county, 2005 29
10. Estimated mining water withdrawals in Colorado by county, 2005 32
11. Water withdrawals and consumption for thermoelectric power generation in Colorado by county, 2005 36
12. Instream water use for hydroelectric power generation in Colorado by county, 2005 37
13. Estimated water withdrawals from select aquifers, by county, Colorado, 2004 40
14. Comparison of 2005 Colorado Statewide Water Supply Initiative forecasted population and water demand and U.S. Geological Survey compilation estimates for population, municipal (public-supply) and industrial (combined), and thermoelectric power generation water use 43
15. Comparison of Colorado total withdrawal estimates, by select category, 1985 and 2005 46

Appendix Tables

1-1–1-8. Water withdrawals for:
1-1. Crop irrigation in Colorado by four-digit hydrologic unit code, 2005 54
1-2. Golf course irrigation in Colorado by four-digit hydrologic unit code, 2005 55
1-3. Public-supply and domestic deliveries in Colorado by four-digit hydrologic unit code, 2005 56
1-4. Self-supplied domestic use in Colorado by four-digit hydrologic unit code, 2005 57

1-5. Self-supplied industrial use in Colorado by four-digit hydrologic unit
      code, 2005 57
1-6. Livestock in Colorado by four-digit hydrologic unit code, 2005 58
1-7. Mining in Colorado by four-digit hydrologic unit code, 2005.......................59
1-8. Thermoelectric power generation in Colorado by four-digit hydrologic
      unit code, 2005...60
1-9. Instream water use for hydroelectric power generation in Colorado by
      four-digit hydrologic unit code, 2005 61

Conversion Factors

Multiply	By	To obtain
Area		
square mile (mi^2)	259.0	hectare (ha)
acre	0.004047	square kilometer (km^2)
Volume		
barrel (bbl), (petroleum, 1 barrel=42 gal)	0.1590	cubic meter (m^3)
gallon	3.785	liter (L)
million gallons (Mgal)	3,785	cubic meter (m^3)
acre-foot (acre-ft)	1,233	cubic meter (m^3)
Flow rate		
gallon per day (gal/d)	3.785	liter per day
million gallons per day (Mgal/d)	0.04381	cubic meter per second (m^3/s)
	1.121	thousand acre-feet per year
	0.6944	thousand gallons per minute
	1.3815	million cubic meters per year
billion gallons per day (Bgal/d)	1.3815	million cubic meters per year
thousand acre-feet per year	0.8921	million gallons per day
	0.6195	thousand gallons per minute
	0.003377	million cubic meters per day

Horizontal coordinate information is referenced to the North American Datum of 1983 (NAD 83).

Estimated Withdrawals and Use of Water in Colorado, 2005

By Tamara Ivahnenko and Jennifer L. Flynn

Abstract

The future health and economic welfare of the people and environment of Colorado depend on a continuous supply of fresh water. Detailed, comprehensive information on the use of water from Colorado's diverse surface-water and groundwater resources is important to water managers and planners by providing information they need to quantify current stresses and estimate and plan for future water needs. As part of the U.S. Geological Survey's (USGS) National Water Use Information Program (NWUIP), Statewide water withdrawal and water-use data have been collected or estimated and summarized in this report by county and by four-digit hydrologic unit code for the following seven water-use categories: irrigation (crop and golf course), public supply, self-supplied domestic, self-supplied industrial, livestock, mining, and thermoelectric power generation. A summary for instream water use for hydroelectric power generation also is included. This report is published in cooperation with the Colorado Water Conservation Board.

In 2005, an estimated 13,581.22 million gallons per day (Mgal/d) was withdrawn from groundwater and surface-water sources in Colorado for the seven water-use categories. Withdrawals from surface water represented about 11,035 Mgal/d, or 81.3 percent of the total, whereas withdrawals from groundwater sources represented an estimated 2,546 Mgal/d or 18.7 percent of the total. Irrigation (combined crop and golf course) totaled 12,362.49 Mgal/d or 91 percent of the total water withdrawals in the State of Colorado. Crop irrigation accounted for 99.7 percent (12,321.85 Mgal/d) of the irrigation, whereas the 243 turf golf courses in Colorado accounted for 0.3 percent (40.64 Mgal/d) of the total irrigation water withdrawals. Total withdrawals for the other water-use categories were public supply, 864.17 Mgal/d; self-supplied domestic, 34.43 Mgal/d; self-supplied industrial, 142.44 Mgal/d; livestock, 33.06 Mgal/d; mining, 21.42 Mgal/d (includes both fresh and saline water); and thermoelectric, 123.21 Mgal/d. The counties with the largest total withdrawals (greater than 500 Mgal/d) were Mesa, Weld, Rio Grande, Montrose, Gunnison, and Saguache. Counties with the smallest total withdrawals (less than 5 Mgal/d) were Clear Creek, Gilpin, and San Juan. Four-digit hydrologic unit codes with the greatest withdrawals were 1019 (South Platte River Basin), 1301 (Rio Grande Basin), and 1102 (Arkansas River Basin); the high withdrawal rates were driven by crop irrigation withdrawals. Total instream water use for hydroelectric power generation was 5,253.60 Mgal/d.

Groundwater withdrawals were estimated for 2004 for the bedrock and overlying alluvial aquifers in the Denver Basin for irrigation, public supply, commercial/industrial, household use only, and domestic/livestock water-use categories. Withdrawals were estimated for input into the USGS Denver Basin model by using the equations in the Senate Bill 96-074 groundwater model. The greatest withdrawals were for public supply. The smallest withdrawals were for household-use-only wells. Douglas County had the greatest groundwater withdrawals (183.98 Mgal/d), whereas Broomfield County had the smallest (3.09 Mgal/d). Of the seven Denver Basin aquifers, the Lower Arapahoe aquifer had the greatest total estimated withdrawals (287.11 Mgal/d), with Douglas County having the greatest public-supply withdrawal of any county (95.29 Mgal/d) from this aquifer. The Upper Dawson aquifer was the least used of the Denver Basin aquifers, based on estimated withdrawals of 17.64 Mgal/d.

As part of the Colorado Statewide Water Supply Initiative (SWSI), forecasts of future water demand were made based on information such as population, climate, and then-current (2000) water-use information and did not include the effects of future water conservation. Categories compared between estimates in the SWSI baseline forecasted water demand and the USGS water-use compilation were limited to county population and water use for municipal (public supply)/industrial purposes and self-supplied thermoelectric power generation. Municipal and industrial water uses are separate categories in the USGS compilation; however, these estimates were combined to compare to the SWSI municipal/industrial baseline forecasted values. Comparison of 2005 population estimates between the SWSI forecast and the 2005 USGS compilation showed that 40 of the 64 counties had a difference of less than 5 percent, and 59 of the counties (92 percent) had a difference of less than 10 percent. For the combined municipal and industrial categories, differences for all the counties ranged from 0.1 to 299.28 percent with a median of 37.96 percent. Of the 64 Colorado counties, 48 (75 percent) had a municipal/industrial USGS estimate lower than the SWSI baseline forecasted water demand. Differences between the SWSI forecasted water demand and USGS compilation estimates may be due to increased conservation efforts, which were not included in the water-demand forecasts, and the differing methodology in deriving the forecasted and estimated values.

A generalized comparison of the published 1985 estimates to water withdrawal estimates 20 years later in 2005 can provide some indication of State water-use trends. Estimates of total water withdrawals were compared for the categories of total irrigation (crop and golf course) public supply (including population), self-supplied domestic (including population), self-supplied industrial, livestock, mining, and thermoelectric. Commercial water use was estimated in 1985 but was not compiled in 2005. Total withdrawals for the seven categories compiled in 1985 and 2005 did not differ greatly and indicated an increase of less than 1 percent. A number of water-use categories indicated an increase in water withdrawals in the 20 years from 1985 to 2005, which included public supply, self-supplied domestic, self-supplied industrial, and thermoelectric uses. These water-use categories can be directly linked to population increases and reflect the overall State population growth from 3.2 million in 1985 to 4.7 million in 2005. As a consequence of increased population and the need for more electricity and manufactured and processed goods, water withdrawals for thermoelectric generation increased 12.2 percent and self-supplied industrial increased 18.4 percent between 1985 and 2005. A number of water-use categories decreased between 1985 and 2005, including irrigation, livestock, and mining. Irrigation estimates decreased the least during these 20 years, less than 1 percent; however, irrigated acres decreased by approximately 10 percent. Livestock withdrawals decreased 45.6 percent and mining decreased 76.5 percent. The decrease in mining withdrawals reflects the decrease in the number of active coal and hard-rock mines in Colorado from 150 in 1985, to 20 in 2005.

Introduction

Water is one of Colorado's most valued renewable resources, and a continuing supply of fresh water is essential to the future health and economic welfare of the people and environment of Colorado. Water-use information is not only important to the State of Colorado, but also to the downstream States as well. Colorado is one of four western States that straddle the Continental Divide, and the headwaters of four major river basins—Arkansas, Colorado, Rio Grande, and South Platte—are within the State (fig. 1). Detailed, comprehensive information on the use of water from Colorado's diverse surface-water and groundwater resources is important as drought, increasing population, and inter- and intra-State water policies and requirements for instream flow put increasing stresses on the finite water supplies. Comprehensive, current, and detailed water-use data will provide Colorado water managers and planners with information they need to

quantify current stresses and to estimate and plan for future water needs.

As part of the U.S. Geological Survey's (USGS) National Water Use Information Program (NWUIP), Statewide water-use data have been collected every fifth year since 1950. Water use for Colorado has been published in summaries of national data (Hutson and others, 2004; Solley and others, 1998, 1993, 1988, 1983; Murray and Reeves, 1977, 1972; Murray, 1968; MacKichan and Kammerer, 1961; MacKichan, 1957, 1951); however, the last Colorado-specific report was written for data collected in 1985 (Litke and Appel, 1989). Because the information in the previous water-use report for 1985 is dated, this report was published by the USGS in cooperation with the Colorado Water Conservation Board (CWCB) to provide updated information on estimated withdrawals and use of water in Colorado for 2005.

Purpose and Scope

The purpose of this report is to summarize the estimated amount of water withdrawn and used from Colorado's groundwater and surface-water resources, collected as part of the USGS NWUIP's data collection effort for 2005. Water withdrawals in Colorado are summarized for each of the following categories: irrigation (crop and golf course), public supply, self-supplied domestic, self-supplied industrial, livestock, mining, and thermoelectric power generation. A summary for instream water use for hydroelectric power generation also is included.

Within each category, withdrawal data are presented by source of withdrawal—groundwater, surface water, or reclaimed wastewater. Consumptive-use information within each category is no longer a required element of the NWUIP; therefore, consumptive-use estimates are only provided for crop irrigation, self-supplied domestic, livestock, and thermoelectric categories. Water withdrawal data for each category also are presented by county and by four-digit hydrologic unit code (HUC) (hydrologic subregion) (fig. 1). Counties and selected cities, towns, and geographic features of Colorado are shown in figure 2.

Sources of Data

Water withdrawal data for 2005 were compiled by the USGS from a variety of sources. Population data for Colorado counties were obtained from the U.S. Census Bureau from population data estimated for 2005 (U.S. Census Bureau, 2006) and provided by the NWUIP. A survey requesting population served, number of connections, and quantity of groundwater and surface water withdrawn was sent to the 844 community water systems (CWSs) in cooperation with the Colorado Department of Public Health and Environment (CDPHE). Because of the low return rate of the CWS surveys (41 percent), the December 2005 Safe Drinking Water Information System (SDWIS) database maintained by the

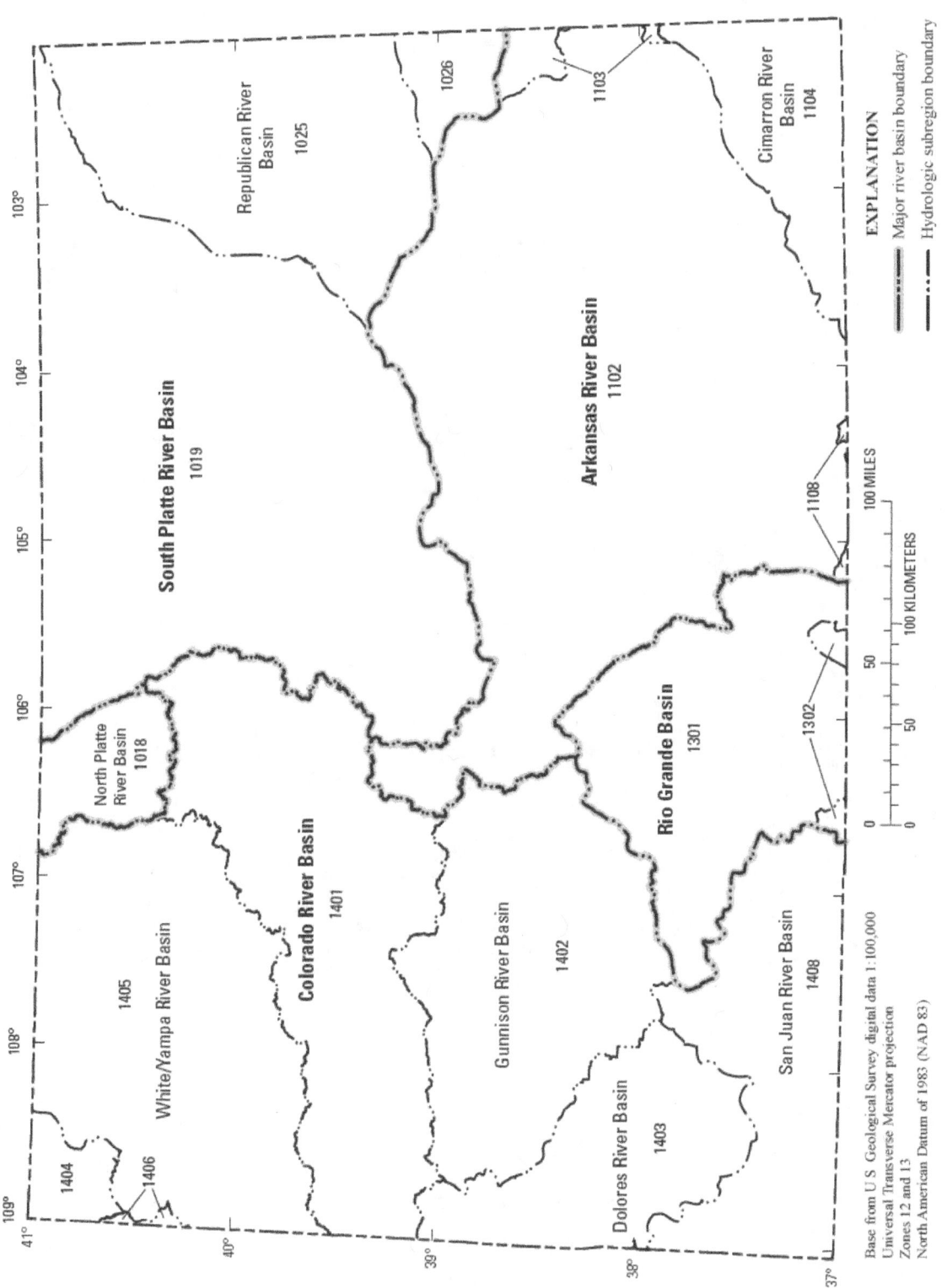

Base from U.S. Geological Survey digital data 1:100,000
Universal Transverse Mercator projection
Zones 12 and 13
North American Datum of 1983 (NAD 83)

Figure 1.   Major river basins and hydrologic unit code numbers in Colorado.

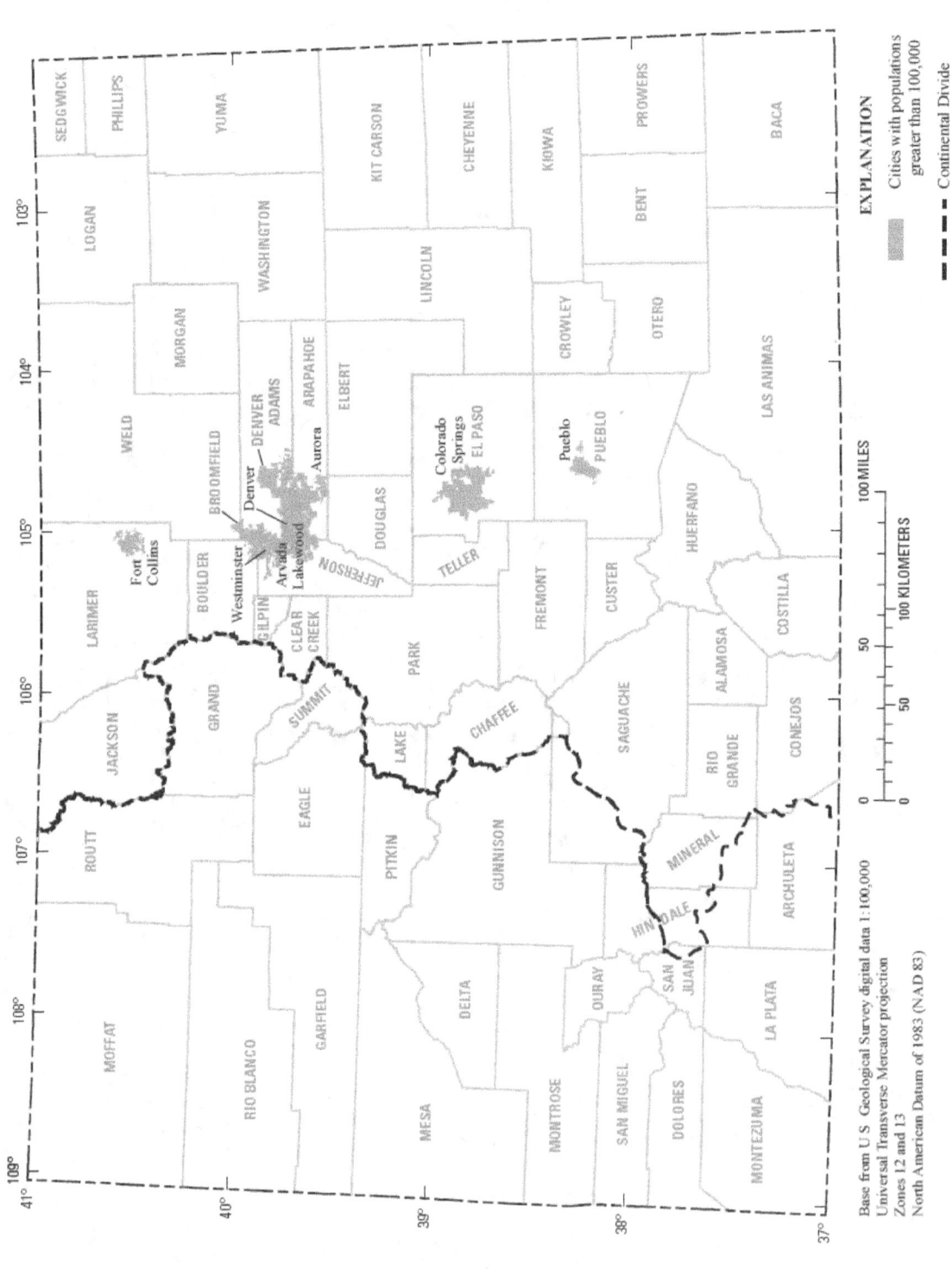

Base from U.S. Geological Survey digital data 1:100,000
Universal Transverse Mercator projection
Zones 12 and 13
North American Datum of 1983 (NAD 83)

Figure 2.   Counties and select cities in Colorado.

U.S. Environmental Protection Agency was used as the estimation basis for the remaining CWSs that did not return a survey. The SDWIS database contained information on whether the public source was groundwater or surface water, whether it was purchased water, and the population served.

Irrigated-acreage data were compiled from a number of sources including the 2002 Agricultural Census (U.S. Department of Agriculture, 2002) and the Colorado Department of Local Affairs (Taxation) (2006). Irrigated-acreage datasets for select basins in 2005, based on aerial surveys and downloadable through the Colorado's Decision Support Systems (CDSS), were not available during the compilation. Geographic information system (GIS) files of Colorado agricultural land used for estimating irrigation water use in HUC basins were based on the USGS National Land Cover Database (2001) (U.S. Geological Survey, 2007). Data for 2005 surface-water diversions and some groundwater pumpage information, by county, was provided by the Colorado Division of Water Resources (CDWR). Water-use estimates for livestock were provided by the NWUIP (Lovelace, 2009a).

Thermoelectric-power-generation data were obtained from the Energy Information Administration (U.S. Department of Energy, 2006), which is the independent statistical and analytical agency within the U.S. Department of Energy. Mining estimates were based on information collected during a telephone survey. Water-use data-request responses were received from 9 of the 12 coal mines, all 4 uranium/vanadium mines, and both gold and gold/silver mines in Colorado. Water use was estimated for the single molybdenum mine in Colorado because no mining water-use information was provided from this operation. Hydroelectric-power and flow data were obtained by direct requests from the Bureau of Reclamation and the various private power utilities.

Limitations of the Data

Every person and most businesses rely on water every day for personal and economic use. It is impossible to collect detailed data for each of these millions of users in the different water-use categories, which entails the need for some degree of estimation. The recommended strategy of the NWUIP, unchanged from 1985, is to collect site-specific water-use data for those large users that account for at least 80 percent of the water use in the category, and estimate the remainder. The resulting database presented in this report is a combination of site-specific and estimated information, and in many categories the estimated information is based on the collected site-specific data. The long-term goal of the NWUIP remains to collect site-specific information whenever possible and refine methods for estimating water-use information.

No precise statements of accuracy of the water withdrawal data can be made because the data were not acquired using rigorous statistical techniques. Generally, the data presented in this report vary in precision from one to three significant figures. Again, unchanged from 1985, groundwater withdrawals for irrigation are among the least accurate of the estimates because those numbers were calculated as a residual in an equation that relied on assumptions of surface-water withdrawals. This is, however, not true for some basins in Colorado. As an example, some irrigation wells in the Arkansas River and South Platte River Basins are metered, providing more accurate pumpage data. Data about withdrawals for public suppliers and golf course irrigation are more accurate because those estimates are based primarily on site-specific information. Powerplant water use (including hydroelectric) and mining information are considered the most accurate data, as these data were collected from nearly complete site-specific telephone surveys.

Methods of Analysis

Amounts of water withdrawn for each category of water use were estimated or calculated by using a variety of methods, which are explained in detail in subsequent sections. Water withdrawals for public supply were obtained from a survey requesting site-specific metered data for some CWSs; however, withdrawals were estimated for those with insufficient information. Survey data were evaluated for reasonableness, and in some cases water purveyors were recontacted to check withdrawal numbers and units for clarity. In general, withdrawals for self-supplied domestic and livestock uses were estimated because these water uses are typically not metered or accurately measured. Water withdrawals for self-supplied industrial uses were based on State diversion information, whereas estimates for thermoelectric and mining uses were based on Federal, State, and telephone survey information.

Estimated Withdrawals and Uses of Water in 2005

The water-use cycle begins with the removal of water from the hydrologic system and ends with the discharge of water to the hydrologic system. There are three basic parts to the cycle: the source (either groundwater or surface water), the use, and the discharge or disposition (for example, return flow and wastewater discharge). Reclaimed wastewater, an additional source water, was documented only for the golf irrigation water-use category; however, reclaimed wastewater in the future may be a more important source water for certain uses (for example, irrigation, thermoelectric cooling water, industrial, and commercial) as water re-use becomes a substantial part of conservation efforts (U.S. Environmental Protection Agency, 2004). For the purposes of this report, it was generally assumed that the water is taken from a source and returned in the same county.

Transmountain diversions and any other anthropogenic structures (pipelines, canals, ditches, and tunnels) designed to move water from one county to another were considered to be part of the natural system. Any water withdrawn solely for the purpose of conveyance or storage was not considered a use and not included in any estimates. However, engineered water diversions have a substantial effect on water flows in Colorado. In 2005, 43 structures (fig. 3, table 1) conveyed a total of 992,123 acre-feet (acre-ft) between the various hydrologic subregions. The largest amount of water was exported from the Colorado River Basin (1401), conveying 468,607 acre-ft primarily to the South Platte (1019) and Arkansas (1102) River Basins.

Water Withdrawals by Category

Water withdrawal information for 2005 was compiled for seven categories: irrigation (crop and golf course), public supply, self-supplied domestic, self-supplied industrial, livestock, mining, and thermoelectric. For each category, surface-water and groundwater withdrawal volumes were compiled and are shown as totals for the State by county (table 2, fig. 4) and by four-digit HUC (table 3). Water withdrawals by category are presented for the hydrologic subregions (hydrologic unit code) in tables 1-1 to 1-9 in the appendix. A summary of instream water use for hydroelectric power generation also was compiled.

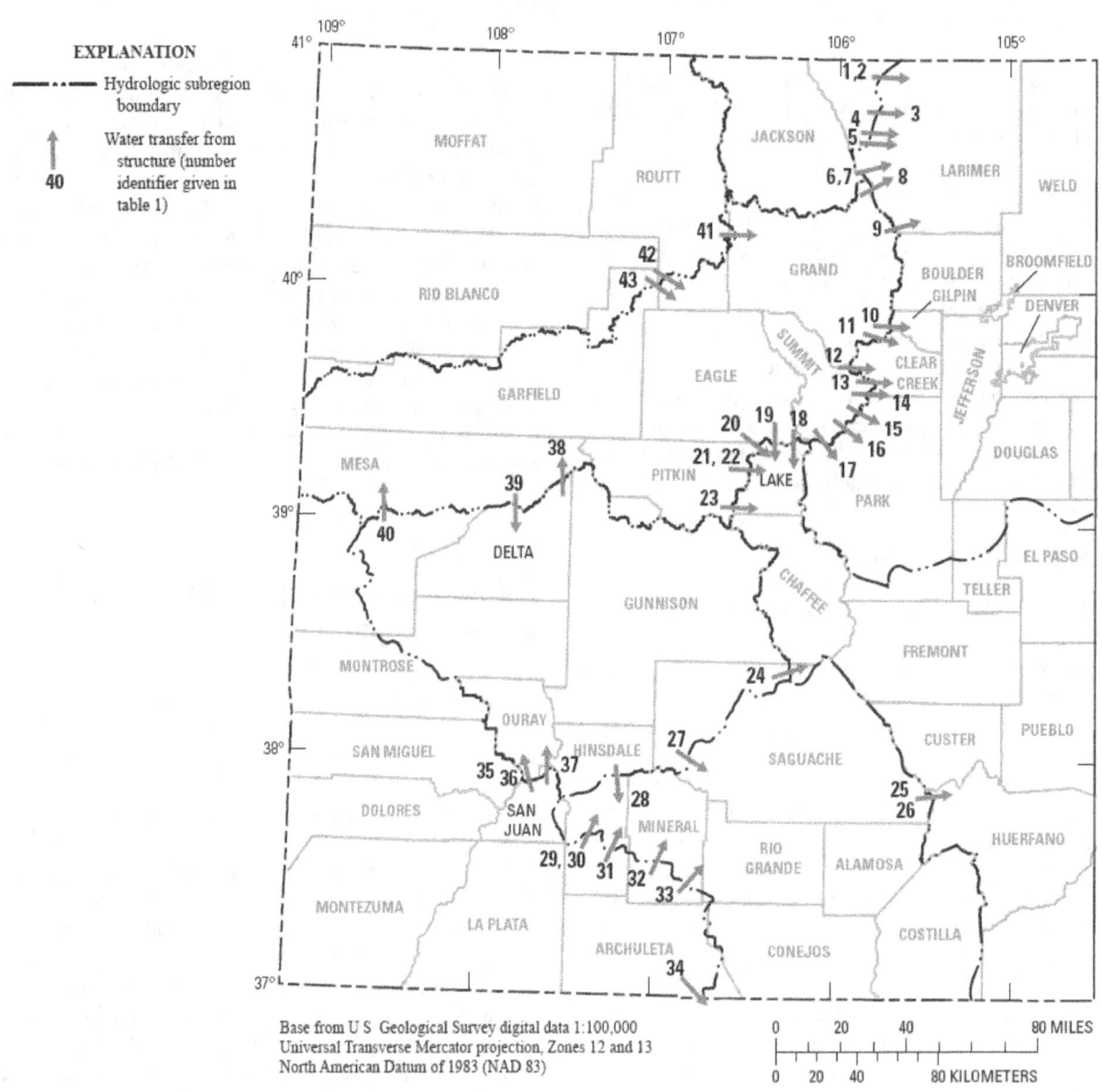

Figure 3.   Interbasin water transfers between hydrologic subregions.

Table 1. Interbasin water transfers between hydrologic subregions, 2005, Colorado.

[Source: Colorado State Engineer's Office; four-digit hydrologic unit code subregions located on figure 1; map numbers located on figure 3]

Map number	Structure	Quantity diverted in 2005 (acre-feet)	Hydrologic unit code From	Hydrologic unit code To
1	Wilson Supply Ditch	3,598	1018	1019
2	Deadman Ditch	1,267	1018	1019
3	Bob Creek Ditch	374	1018	1019
4	Laramie-Poudre Tunnel	18,211	1018	1019
5	Skyline Ditch	0	1018	1019
6	Cameron Pass Ditch	178	1018	1019
7	Michigan Ditch	5,983	1018	1019
8	Grand River Ditch	21,171	1401	1019
9	Alva B. Adams Tunnel	162,912	1401	1019
10	Moffat Water Tunnel	56,273	1401	1019
11	Berthoud Pass Ditch	408	1401	1019
12	Straight Creek Tunnel	361	1401	1019
13	Vidler Tunnel	517	1401	1019
14	Harold D. Roberts Tunnel	59,233	1401	1019
15	Columbine Ditch	0	1401	1019
16	Boreas Pass Ditch	133	1401	1019
17	Hoosier Pass Tunnel	10,036	1401	1019
18	Ewing Ditch	784	1401	1102
19	Warren E. Wurts Ditch	2,298	1401	1102
20	Homestake Tunnel	42,818	1401	1102
21	FryArk Project Boustead Tunnel	55,351	1401	1102
22	Ivanhoe Tunnel	4931	1401	1102
23	Twin Lakes Tunnel	51,382	1401	1102
24	Larkspur Ditch	174	1401	1102
25	Hudson Branch Ditch	879	1301	1102
26	Medano Ditch	845	1301	1102
27	Tarbell Ditch	1,121	1402	1301
28	Tabor Ditch No. 2	1,079	1402	1301
29	Weminuche Pass Ditch	2,706	1408	1301
30	Pine River-Weminuche Pass Ditch	474	1408	1301
31	Williams Squaw Pass Ditch	632	1408	1301
32	Don La Font Ditches 1 and 2	53	1408	1301
33	Treasure Pass Diversion Ditch	337	1408	1301

Table 1.   Interbasin water transfers between hydrologic subregions, 2005, Colorado.—Continued

[Source: Colorado State Engineer's Office; four-digit hydrologic unit code subregions located on figure 1; map numbers located on figure 3]

Map number	Structure	Quantity diverted in 2005 (acre-feet)	Hydrologic unit code	
			From	To
34	San Juan Chama Project (Azotea Tunnel)	155,195	1408	1302
35	Red Mountain Ditch	38	1408	1402
36	Carbon Lake Ditch	0	1408	1402
37	Mineral Point Ditch	0	1408	1402
38	Divide Creek Highline Feeder Ditch	441	1402	1401
39	Leon Tunnel	100	1401	1402
40	Redlands Power Canal	327,654	1402	1401
41	Sarvis Creek Ditch	561	1405	1401
42	Stillwater Ditch	1515	1405	1401
43	Dome Creek Ditch	100	1405	1401
Total		992,123		

In 2005, an estimated 13,581.22 million gallons per day (Mgal/d) was withdrawn from groundwater and surface-water sources in Colorado for the seven water-use categories (excluding hydroelectric power generation) (table 2, fig. 4). Withdrawals from surface water represented about 11,035 Mgal/d, or 81.3 percent of the total, whereas withdrawals from groundwater sources represented an estimated 2,546 Mgal/d or 18.7 percent of the total. Irrigation withdrawals (combined crop and golf course) totaled 12,362.49 Mgal/d or 91 percent of the total water withdrawals in the State of Colorado. Crop irrigation accounted for 99.7 percent (12,321.85 Mgal/d) of the irrigation withdrawals, whereas the 243 turf golf courses in Colorado used 0.3 percent (40.64 Mgal/d) of the total irrigation water withdrawals.

Total withdrawals for the other water-use categories were public supply, 864.17 Mgal/d; self-supplied industrial, 142.44 Mgal/d; self-supplied domestic, 34.43 Mgal/d; livestock, 33.06 Mgal/d; mining, 21.42 Mgal/d (includes both fresh and saline water), and thermoelectric, 123.21 Mgal/d. The counties with the largest total withdrawals (greater than 500 Mgal/d), were Mesa, Weld, Rio Grande, Montrose, Gunnison, and Saguache. Counties with the smallest total withdrawals (less than 5 Mgal/d) were Clear Creek, Gilpin, and San Juan (table 2). Four-digit HUCs with the greatest withdrawals were 1019 (South Platte River Basin), 1301 (Rio Grande Basin), and 1102 (Arkansas River Basin); the high withdrawal rates were driven by crop irrigation withdrawals (table 3; fig. 5).

Table 2. Total population and water withdrawals in Colorado by county, 2005.

[Mgal/d, million gallons per day; acre-ft/yr, acre feet per year; values may not add for totals due to rounding]

County (fig. 2)	Population of county (thousands)	Withdrawals by category (Mgal/d)								Total withdrawals (Mgal/d)	Total withdrawals (thousand acre-ft/yr)
		Irrigation (crop)	Irrigation (golf course)	Public-supply	Domestic	Industrial	Livestock	Mining	Thermo-electric		
Adams	399.43	120.17	1.93	51.07	0.02	2.44	0.22	0.17	9.25	185.27	207.69
Alamosa	15.28	267.68	.08	2.00	.53	.00	.13	.01	.00	270.43	303.15
Arapahoe	529.09	5.23	3.34	75.68	.51	.01	.12	.03	.00	84.92	95.20
Archuleta	11.89	69.83	.22	.77	.47	.00	.09	.10	.00	71.48	80.13
Baca	4.07	144.86	.00	.75	.10	.00	.74	.33	.00	146.78	164.54
Bent	5.56	209.17	.11	1.13	.13	.00	.73	.06	.00	211.33	236.90
Boulder	280.44	149.86	1.54	45.62	.25	.41	.18	.05	5.82	203.73	228.38
Broomfield	43.48	.00	.24	4.45	.54	.00	.00	.00	.00	5.23	5.86
Chaffee	16.97	103.41	.19	1.69	.31	.00	.08	.05	.00	105.73	118.52
Cheyenne	1.95	37.95	.11	.42	.18	.02	.21	.36	.00	39.25	44.00
Clear Creek	9.20	0.00	.00	1.30	.26	.07	.00	.01	.00	1.64	1.84
Conejos	8.51	345.23	.00	.87	.57	.00	.29	.03	.00	346.99	388.98
Costilla	3.42	172.34	.00	.43	.12	.00	.09	.03	.00	173.01	193.94
Crowley	5.40	33.05	.00	.79	.07	.00	.33	.02	.00	34.26	38.41
Custer	3.86	44.79	.01	.12	.31	.00	.06	.03	.00	45.32	50.80
Delta	29.95	450.61	.51	5.89	1.93	.23	.40	.62	.00	460.19	515.87
Denver	557.92	.00	1.44	228.53	.00	4.21	.00	.00	2.26	236.44	265.05
Dolores	1.83	34.24	.00	.32	.12	.00	.03	.03	.00	34.74	38.94
Douglas	249.42	10.60	1.49	30.16	.96	.01	.12	.03	.00	43.37	48.62
Eagle	47.53	143.91	3.34	9.19	.01	.26	.08	.04	.00	156.83	175.81
Elbert	22.79	33.11	.21	1.05	1.68	.00	.47	.11	.00	36.63	41.06
El Paso	565.58	31.90	2.33	116.66	3.25	.00	.35	.05	2.54	157.08	176.09
Fremont	47.77	125.62	.98	7.60	.38	.49	.18	.12	15.48	150.85	169.10
Garfield	49.81	332.02	1.61	14.62	1.15	.50	.27	.07	.00	350.24	392.62

Table 2. Total population and water withdrawals in Colorado by county, 2005.—Continued

[Mgal/d, million gallons per day; acre-ft/yr, acre feet per year; values may not add for totals due to rounding]

County (fig. 2)	Population of county (thousands)	Withdrawals by category (Mgal/d)								Total withdrawals (Mgal/d)	Total withdrawals (thousand acre-ft/yr)
		Irrigation (crop)	Irrigation (golf course)	Public-supply	Domestic	Industrial	Livestock	Mining	Thermo-electric		
Gilpin	4.93	0.00	0.00	0.51	0.11	0.00	0.00	0.00	0.00	0.62	0.70
Grand	13.21	226.17	.43	2.39	.07	1.39	.16	.06	.00	230.67	258.58
Gunnison	14.23	550.78	.30	2.83	.03	.67	.17	.29	.00	555.07	622.23
Hinsdale	.77	69.75	.00	.51	.06	.00	.02	.01	.00	70.35	78.86
Huerfano	7.77	35.11	.29	.85	.04	.00	.12	.09	.00	36.50	40.92
Jackson	1.45	427.76	.00	.18	.12	.02	.25	.19	.00	428.52	480.37
Jefferson	526.80	27.50	4.51	9.63	5.71	39.38	.06	.03	.03	86.85	97.36
Kiowa	1.45	18.03	.11	.14	.04	.00	.22	.07	.00	18.57	20.82
Kit Carson	7.64	281.00	.21	1.51	.42	.00	1.47	.13	.01	284.75	319.20
Lake	7.74	12.69	.03	1.13	.25	.14	.00	.15	.00	14.39	16.13
La Plata	47.45	368.61	.84	5.22	.39	.44	.26	.33	.00	376.09	421.60
Larimer	271.93	418.87	2.76	56.73	.29	3.36	.92	.51	.00	483.44	541.94
Las Animas	15.45	62.47	.00	2.40	.81	.00	.44	1.55	.00	67.67	75.86
Lincoln	5.62	14.79	.11	.81	.10	.00	.48	.12	.00	16.41	18.40
Logan	20.72	284.23	.38	2.54	.43	.00	2.28	.56	.00	290.42	325.56
Mesa	129.87	864.45	1.89	14.58	.20	.55	.57	.21	43.85	926.30	1,038.38
Mineral	.93	21.92	.00	.27	.18	.00	.01	.01	.00	22.39	25.10
Moffat	13.42	139.95	.45	1.60	.44	.00	.45	1.12	12.81	156.82	175.80
Montezuma	24.78	246.46	.21	2.59	.05	.05	.23	.06	.00	249.65	279.86
Montrose	37.48	679.13	1.24	8.87	.36	1.77	.62	.62	1.68	694.29	778.30
Morgan	27.99	279.77	.38	6.16	.28	.91	2.96	.30	3.94	294.70	330.36
Otero	19.50	387.40	.19	5.07	.05	.00	.70	.06	.00	393.47	441.08
Ouray	4.26	102.90	.21	.49	.17	.00	.08	.02	.00	103.87	116.44
Park	16.95	19.32	.00	.34	1.57	.56	.10	.07	.00	21.96	24.62

Table 2. Total population and water withdrawals in Colorado by county, 2005.—Continued

[Mgal/d, million gallons per day; acre-ft/yr, acre feet per year; values may not add for totals due to rounding]

| County (fig. 2) | Population of county (thousands) | Withdrawals by category (Mgal/d) | | | | | | | | Total withdrawals (Mgal/d) | Total withdrawals (thousand acre-ft/yr) |
		Irrigation (crop)	Irrigation (golf course)	Public-supply	Domestic	Industrial	Livestock	Mining	Thermo-electric		
Phillips	4.59	121.51	0.22	1.66	0.50	0.00	0.53	0.07	0.00	124.49	139.55
Pitkin	14.79	126.22	.24	4.38	.02	.00	.02	.01	.00	130.89	146.73
Prowers	13.89	484.16	.00	1.80	.47	.25	1.22	.11	.00	488.01	547.06
Pueblo	151.32	123.88	.82	83.92	.57	72.32	.39	.12	18.88	300.90	337.31
Rio Blanco	5.97	226.94	.30	1.22	.35	2.33	.28	9.92	.00	241.34	270.54
Rio Grande	12.23	727.11	.15	1.40	.82	.00	.15	.06	.00	729.69	817.98
Routt	21.31	188.59	1.21	4.55	.78	3.01	.34	.59	2.52	201.59	225.98
Saguache	7.03	506.76	.11	.78	.45	.00	.29	.06	.00	508.45	569.97
San Juan	.58	.00	.00	.06	.02	.18	.00	.01	.00	.27	.30
San Miguel	7.21	27.27	.08	.75	.14	.00	.09	.04	.00	28.37	31.80
Sedgwick	2.53	98.42	.11	.63	.15	.00	.38	.02	.00	99.71	111.77
Summit	24.89	59.05	.49	6.06	.34	.02	.03	.01	.00	66.00	73.99
Teller	21.92	3.46	.21	1.32	.15	1.21	.03	.04	.00	6.42	7.20
Washington	4.63	118.37	.05	.69	.28	.00	.67	.59	.00	120.65	135.25
Weld	228.94	725.30	2.33	24.42	2.54	5.23	7.12	.68	4.14	771.76	865.14
Yuma	9.79	390.17	.10	2.07	.83	.00	3.78	.18	.00	397.13	445.18
Total	4,665.18	12,321.85	40.64	864.17	34.43	142.44	33.06	21.42	123.21	13,581.22	15,224.55

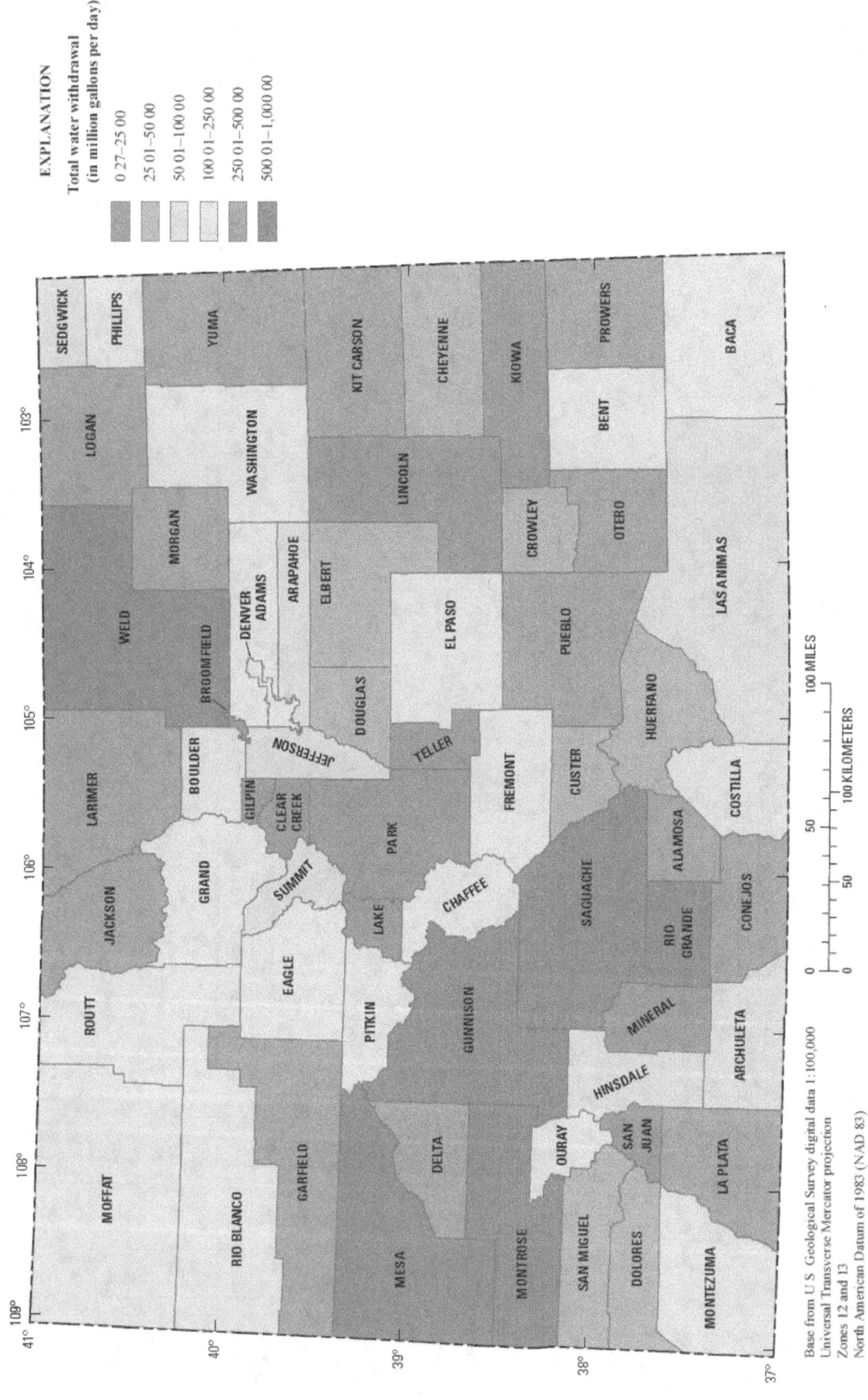

Base from U.S. Geological Survey digital data 1:100,000
Universal Transverse Mercator projection
Zones 12 and 13
North American Datum of 1983 (NAD 83)

Figure 4. Estimated total water withdrawals by Colorado county, 2005.

Table 3. Total population and water withdrawals in Colorado by hydrologic unit code, 2005.

[Mgal/d, million gallons per day; acre-ft/yr, acre feet per year; values may not add for totals due to rounding]

Hydrologic unit code (fig. 1)	Population of hydrologic unit code (thousands)	Withdrawals by category (Mgal/d)								Total withdrawals (Mgal/d)	Total withdrawals (thousand acre-ft/yr)
		Irrigation (crop)	Irrigation (golf course)	Public-supply	Domestic	Industrial	Livestock	Mining	Thermo-electric		
1018	1.45	458.49	0.00	56.91	0.12	0.02	0.39	0.19	.00	516.12	578.57
1019	3,208.08	1,994.23	21.86	602.83	16.19	57.22	14.27	2.84	25.44	2,734.87	3,065.79
1025	26.33	1,011.25	.59	3.98	1.15	0.0	6.80	.72	.01	1,024.49	1,148.46
1026	1.54	72.75	.11	.33	.15	.02	.27	.20	0.0	73.83	82.76
1102	874.26	1,590.25	4.18	106.73	7.01	73.79	5.93	2.79	36.90	1,827.58	2,048.72
1103	.60	22.76	.00	.00	.02	0.0	.07	.02	0.0	22.87	25.64
1104	4.07	228.70	.00	.75	.11	0.0	.17	.34	0.0	230.08	257.92
1108	.00	.00	.00	.00	.00	.00	.00	.00	.00	.00	.00
1301	47.41	1,966.09	.34	5.74	2.72	0.0	.86	.20	0.0	1,975.93	2,215.02
1302	.10	41.95	.00	.01	.00	0.0	.02	0.0	0.0	41.98	47.06
1401	274.24	1,701.75	8.00	58.60	1.81	2.71	.87	.39	43.85	1,817.98	2,037.96
1402	90.42	1,790.65	2.26	15.76	2.40	2.49	1.16	1.10	0.0	1,815.82	2,035.53
1403	12.13	170.59	.08	3.43	.19	0.18	.55	.52	1.68	177.22	198.67
1404	.04	.42	.00	0.00	.00	0.0	.07	0.0	0.0	.50	.56
1405	39.81	545.47	1.96	2.82	1.53	5.34	.98	11.63	15.33	585.06	655.85
1406	.02	.20	.00	0.0	.00	0.0	.01	0.0	0.0	.21	.24
1408	84.71	726.31	1.28	6.28	1.03	.67	.65	.48	.00	736.69	825.83
Total	4,665.18	12,321.85	40.64	864.17	34.43	142.44	33.06	21.42	123.21	13,581.22	15,224.55

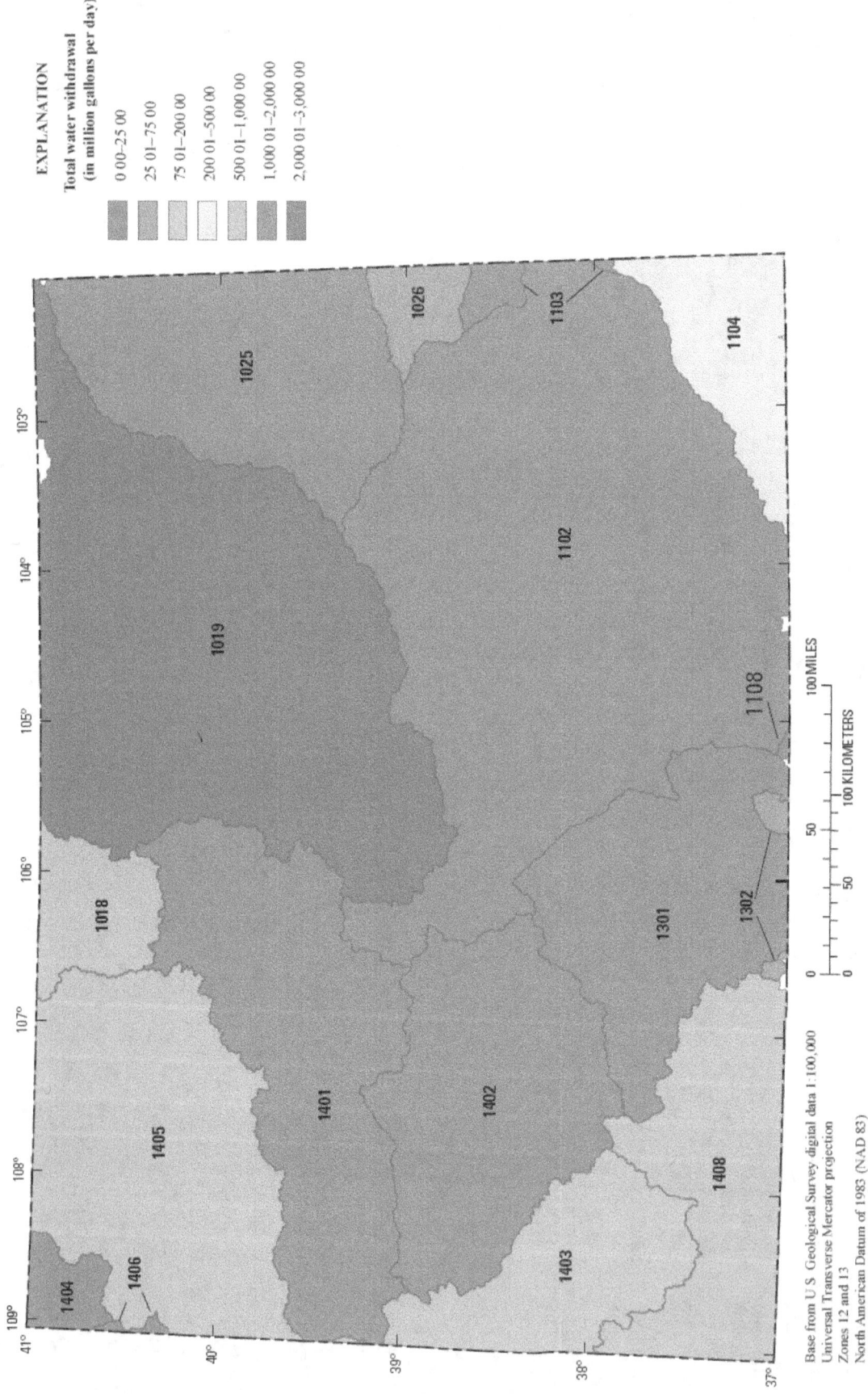

EXPLANATION

Total water withdrawal
(in million gallons per day)

0 00–25 00

25 01–75 00

75 01–200 00

200 01–500 00

500 01–1,000 00

1,000 01–2,000 00

2,000 01–3,000 00

Base from U S Geological Survey digital data 1 100,000
Universal Transverse Mercator projection
Zones 12 and 13
North American Datum of 1983 (NAD 83)

Figure 5.   Estimated total water withdrawals by four-digit hydrologic unit codes, Colorado, 2005.

Irrigation

Irrigation water use includes all water that is applied to farm, orchard, vegetable, pasture, and horticultural crops to promote growth, ensure germination, prevent frost damage, and help in crop cooling or in harvesting and dust suppression. Water application is not evenly distributed throughout the year, but most intensely applied during the growing season. Irrigation water use also includes water to maintain recreational areas such as parks, landscaping, and public and private golf courses. All water for crop irrigation is considered self-supplied, whereas golf course irrigation may be a mixture of self-supplied, reclaimed wastewater, or public supply.

Crop irrigation water use was calculated on the basis of county irrigated acreage for alfalfa, dry beans, corn (grain and silage), sorghum, barley, and wheat (U.S. Department of Agriculture, 2006), and orchards, oats, potatoes, soybeans, sunflowers, sugarbeets, vegetables, and hay/forage (U.S. Department of Agriculture, 2002). Irrigated acres by type of irrigation system (flood, sprinkler, and microirrigation) were obtained from tax records through the Colorado Department of Local Affairs (2006) (flood and sprinkler) and the CDWR (microirrigation). Irrigated-acreage datasets from the CDSS were not utilized for the 2005 compilation because the datasets for select basins in 2005, based on aerial surveys, were not available during the compilation. Datasets of irrigated acreage for the Colorado River Basin were available from 2001, and information for select counties in the Arkansas River Basin were available from 2003. Because much of the irrigated acreage data for the State was temporally inconsistent for 2005, the U.S. Department of Agriculture irrigated-acreage dataset was used instead for the compilation. Surface-water diversions and some groundwater withdrawal information (predominantly wells in the South Platte River and Arkansas River Basins) were obtained through the CDSS, Water Use Data—HydroBase (Colorado Water Conservation Board and Colorado Division of Water Resources, 2006). The remaining groundwater withdrawals were estimated by subtracting the surface-water withdrawals from the net irrigation-water requirement (crop consumptive use calculated using the Blaney-Criddle formula (Blaney and others, 1952) minus effective precipitation); the net irrigation-water requirement was calculated using the program StateCU, a product of the CDSS (Colorado Water Conservation Board and Colorado Division of Water Resources, 2006). StateCU is a modified version of the U.S. Bureau of Reclamation XCONS2 program that uses climate station data and the Blaney-Criddle formula to calculate net irrigation-water requirements for alfalfa and pasture grass at climate station locations throughout the State. The input files for StateCU were updated with 2005 temperature, precipitation, and frost data from HydroBase, and simulations of irrigation requirements for 133 climate stations were made. From these, one climate station was chosen to represent conditions in each county.

To determine an irrigation-water requirement for a specific crop, a crop coefficient (obtained from the Colorado State University Extension Service, 2006) was multiplied by the irrigation water requirement for the index crop. The median crop coefficients for orchards and vegetables were obtained from an internal input file in StateCU. For stations where the index crop was grass pasture, a conversion factor of 1.11 was multiplied with the crop coefficient to be equivalent to alfalfa. To calculate the irrigation-water requirement, the crop and county specific irrigation-water requirement was multiplied by the number of acres of each crop in each county for a total irrigation-water requirement and converted to acre-feet. This value was subtracted from the surface-water irrigation-diversion information provided by the CDWR to determine the irrigation groundwater withdrawals and converted to million gallons per day. Groundwater data were checked with county extension agents and previous compilation information for availability of the resource, especially in counties where the calculated irrigation-water requirement was much less than the surface-water diversions provided by CDWR.

Finally, in some counties, data checks were needed because irrigation withdrawals were initially estimated to be greater than 10 acre-ft per irrigated acre. In discussions with ditch company managers and district water commissioners, some surface-water diversion information may have been overestimated, or included a large error. Irrigation withdrawal estimates were recalculated based on provided information and were less than the 10 acre-ft per irrigated acre. Future compilations of irrigation water use can include CDSS and Hydrobase datasets, such as satellite imagery of irrigated croplands, crop consumptive use, and water rights, which will enable a more comprehensive method to estimate water use.

Irrigation (crop and golf course) accounted for the largest withdrawals in Colorado (12,362.49 Mgal/d), which includes water applied to crops as well as water lost through conveyances. Approximately 91 percent of the total water withdrawn in Colorado in 2005 was for the irrigation process, and 81 percent (10,004.67 Mgal/d) of the irrigation water was supplied from surface-water sources. Irrigated land (both crop and pasture) totaled 2,998,480 acres and had 12,321.85 Mgal/d of water withdrawn for irrigation. Mesa, Weld, and Rio Grande Counties each accounted for about 6 to 7 percent of the total crop irrigation withdrawals (table 4). Mesa, Weld, Rio Grande, Montrose, Saguache, and Gunnison Counties had the largest irrigation withdrawals (more than 500 Mgal/d), and with the exception of the Arkansas River Basin, the other major river basins in Colorado have a county or number of counties that have an irrigation withdrawal greater than 500 Mgal/d (fig. 6). Consumptive use is estimated to be 55.1 percent of the total withdrawals for irrigation (table 4), and the average annual consumptive-use rate for irrigated acres was about 2.54 acre-ft per irrigated acre.

As part of the 2005 water-use compilation, golf course irrigation information was collected through a Web-based survey sponsored by the Rocky Mountain Golf Course Superintendents Association (RMGCSA) (Ivahnenko, 2009). Of the 243 turf golf courses in Colorado, 237 golf courses had superintendents as members of the RMGCSA, and 101 surveys (43 percent) were returned (both electronically and by telephone) from the superintendents. At least one golf course survey was returned in nearly every county in which a golf course is located (the exceptions are Chaffee, Elbert, Montezuma, Ouray, Prowers, Teller, Saguache, and Sedgwick Counties). Golf course irrigation totaled 40.64 Mgal/d, and had an estimated 2.27 acre-ft per irrigated course acre. Most of the withdrawals were from surface-water sources (32.92 Mgal/d), with less than 20 percent from groundwater sources (7.72 Mgal/d). Additional detailed analysis of golf-course water withdrawals are reported in Ivahnenko (2009).

Table 4. Estimated crop irrigation water withdrawals in Colorado by county, 2005.

[Mgal/d, million gallons per day; acre-ft/yr, acre feet per year ; values may not add for totals due to rounding]

County (fig. 2)	Irrigated acres, by type (thousand acres)			Withdrawals by source (Mgal/d)		Consumptive use (Mgal/d)	Withdrawals by source (thousand acre-ft/yr)		Consumptive use (thousand acre-ft/yr)
	Flood	Sprinkler	Micro	Groundwater	Surface water		Groundwater	Surface water	
Adams	13.54	15.29	0.00	1.32	118.85	49.28	1.48	133.23	55.24
Alamosa	39.35	73.14	.00	228.49	39.19	255.84	256.14	43.93	286.79
Arapahoe	.00	1.75	.00	1.69	3.54	4.10	1.89	3.97	4.60
Archuleta	16.34	.00	.00	1.33	68.50	16.93	1.49	76.79	18.98
Baca	16.86	69.11	.00	144.73	.13	125.86	162.42	.15	141.09
Bent	59.10	.00	.00	6.88	143.33	143.33	7.71	226.77	160.67
Boulder	36.72	.00	.00	.04	149.82	62.51	.04	167.95	70.08
Broomfield	.00	.00	.00	.00	.00	.00	.00	.00	.00
Chaffee	15.42	3.80	.00	.02	103.39	43.83	.02	115.90	49.13
Cheyenne	2.18	23.22	.00	37.66	.29	34.03	42.22	.33	38.15
Clear Creek	.00	.00	.00	.00	.00	.00	.00	.00	.00
Conejos	69.87	29.46	.00	6.88	338.35	228.49	7.71	379.29	256.13
Costilla	22.59	22.59	.00	42.56	129.78	108.36	47.71	145.48	121.47
Crowley	16.44	.00	.00	3.76	29.29	22.65	4.21	32.83	25.39
Custer	24.79	.00	.00	.09	44.70	40.64	.10	50.11	45.56
Delta	48.68	.00	.00	.01	450.60	133.02	.01	505.12	149.12
Denver	.00	.00	.00	.00	.00	.00	.00	.00	.00
Dolores	1.63	6.73	.00	4.02	30.22	14.27	4.51	33.88	16.00
Douglas	2.71	1.70	.00	2.19	8.41	6.64	2.45	9.43	7.44
Eagle	19.64	.00	.00	.27	143.64	34.81	.30	161.02	39.02
Elbert	.82	4.46	.00	1.21	31.90	8.47	1.36	35.76	9.50
El Paso	4.41	6.22	.00	5.32	26.58	21.59	5.96	29.80	24.20
Fremont	15.79	.00	.00	.21	125.41	35.52	.24	140.58	39.82
Garfield	50.30	.00	.00	.16	331.86	58.47	.18	372.02	65.55

Table 4. Estimated crop irrigation water withdrawals in Colorado by county, 2005.—Continued

[Mgal/d, million gallons per day; acre-ft/yr, acre feet per year ; values may not add for totals due to rounding]

County (fig. 2)	Irrigated acres, by type (thousand acres)			Withdrawals by source (Mgal/d)		Consumptive use (Mgal/d)	Withdrawals by source (thousand acre-ft/yr)		Consumptive use (thousand acre-ft/yr)
	Flood	Sprinkler	Micro	Ground-water	Surface water		Ground-water	Surface water	
Gilpin	0.00	0.00	0.00	0.00	0.00	0.00	0.00	0.00	0.00
Grand	30.36	.00	.00	.00	226.17	84.12	.00	253.54	94.30
Gunnison	41.48	.00	.00	.46	550.32	132.36	.52	616.91	148.37
Hinsdale	5.33	.00	.00	.05	69.70	10.73	.06	78.13	12.03
Huerfano	16.93	.00	.00	.00	35.11	25.22	.00	39.36	28.27
Jackson	114.41	.00	.00	2.13	425.63	191.31	2.39	477.13	214.46
Jefferson	4.36	.00	.00	.13	27.37	9.43	.15	30.68	10.57
Kiowa	3.31	1.30	.00	6.52	1.51	6.88	7.31	1.69	7.71
Kit Carson	11.14	151.68	.00	280.58	.42	238.01	314.53	.47	266.81
Lake	1.80	.00	.00	.03	12.66	.38	.03	14.19	.43
La Plata	54.72	.00	.00	.68	367.93	128.67	.76	412.45	144.24
Larimer	83.01	.00	.00	60.64	358.23	155.06	67.98	401.58	173.82
Las Animas	24.89	.00	.00	.06	62.41	48.73	.07	69.96	54.62
Lincoln	1.25	3.35	.00	13.22	1.57	4.74	14.82	1.76	5.32
Logan	73.95	29.69	.00	2.65	281.58	255.99	2.97	315.65	286.96
Mesa	85.01	.00	.00	.23	864.22	191.30	.26	968.79	214.45
Mineral	2.06	.00	.00	.61	21.31	3.66	.68	23.89	4.10
Moffat	18.35	2.17	.00	.84	139.11	57.94	.94	155.94	64.95
Montezuma	44.30	15.95	.00	.10	246.36	189.98	.11	276.17	212.96
Montrose	96.29	.00	.00	.73	678.40	268.12	.82	760.49	300.56
Morgan	56.33	88.56	.00	104.69	177.08	244.74	115.12	198.51	274.35
Otero	63.77	.00	3.0	17.21	370.19	209.93	19.29	414.98	235.33
Ouray	14.53	.00	.00	.13	102.77	37.67	.15	115.21	42.23
Park	30.26	.00	.00	.00	19.32	17.37	.00	21.66	19.47
Phillips	3.48	63.28	.00	121.51	.00	94.53	136.21	.00	105.97
Pitkin	13.29	.00	.00	.00	126.22	18.72	.00	141.49	20.98
Prowers	112.14	16.80	.16	27.45	456.71	314.70	30.77	511.97	352.78
Pueblo	28.03	2.04	.00	8.68	115.20	105.54	9.73	129.14	118.31
Rio Blanco	47.53	.00	.00	3.67	223.27	115.38	4.11	250.29	129.22
Rio Grande	64.98	70.71	.00	196.44	530.67	334.23	220.21	594.88	374.67
Routt	52.22	.00	.00	5.40	183.19	88.63	6.05	205.36	99.35
Saguache	118.60	.00	.00	350.52	156.24	479.84	392.93	175.15	537.90

Table 4.   Estimated crop irrigation water withdrawals in Colorado by county, 2005.—Continued

[Mgal/d, million gallons per day; acre-ft/yr, acre feet per year ; values may not add for totals due to rounding]

County (fig. 2)	Irrigated acres, by type (thousand acres)			Withdrawals by source (Mgal/d)		Consumptive use (Mgal/d)	Withdrawals by source (thousand acre-ft/yr)		Consumptive use (thousand acre-ft/yr)
	Flood	Sprinkler	Micro	Ground-water	Surface water		Ground-water	Surface water	
San Juan	0.00	0.00	0.00	0.00	0.00	0.00	0.00	0.00	0.00
San Miguel	9.92	.00	.00	.00	27.27	26.78	.00	30.57	30.02
Sedgwick	20.85	27.23	.00	56.40	42.02	92.16	63.22	47.10	110.22
Summit	5.85	.00	.00	.00	59.05	8.63	.00	66.20	9.67
Teller	.61	.00	.00	.00	3.46	3.36	.00	3.88	3.76
Washington	7.17	41.28	.00	.00	6.13	110.29	125.82	6.87	123.63
Weld	24.87	83.73	.00	.00	717.27	702.67	121.10	691.96	787.70
Yuma	8.14	260.40	.00	.00	8.97	327.05	427.33	10.06	366.62
Total	1,872.52	1,122.80	3.16	2,350.07	9,971.78	6,783.49	2,634.43	11,178.37	7,604.29

Public Supply

Public supply is water supplied by a publicly or privately owned water system for public distribution, sometimes also known as a "municipal-supply system" or "community water system" (CWS). Any water system that serves drinking water to at least 25 people for at least 60 days of the calendar year or has at least 15 service connections is considered a public-supply system (U.S. Environmental Protection Agency, 2009). In addition to providing water to domestic customers, CWSs also deliver water to commercial, industrial, and thermoelectric power users. In 2005, there were 844 CWSs in Colorado, including three tribal systems (U.S. Environmental Protection Agency, 2006). These tribal systems served an estimated population of 4,420 and are included in the county public-supply water-use estimates.

A water-use survey, in cooperation with the Colorado Department of Public Health and Environment, was distributed by mail to the 844 CWSs. These surveys requested information about source of water, name of aquifer, quantity of water withdrawn, population served, number of service connections, water purchased, water sold, quantity of water delivered to each type of customer (domestic, industrial, and commercial), and water system loss. Of the 844 surveys sent, 41 percent were returned. No surveys were returned for Ouray and San Juan Counties. Counties in which all CWSs returned surveys were Cheyenne, Hinsdale, Jackson, Mineral, and Rio Blanco. Of the nine very large water systems, those systems serving more than 100,000 people (U.S. Environmental Protection Agency, 2006) in the State, eight returned information. An estimated 75 percent of the population served by public-supply systems and 73 percent of the total water

delivered were accounted for through the CWSs that did return the survey.

For the remaining CWSs, groundwater and surface-water withdrawals were estimated on the basis of the population served and multiplied by a county water-use coefficient. The population served was based on the purveyor reported information in the 2005 U.S. Environmental Protection Agency's SDWIS database (U.S. Environmental Protection Agency, 2006), corrected to the U.S. Census Bureau's county population data (U.S. Census Bureau, 2006). The SDWIS database also contains basic information on source water (whether groundwater or surface water) for the CWSs, including information on which systems have purchased water. The county coefficient was based on the information returned in the site-specific survey and ranged from 22 to 850 gallons per day (gal/d) per capita. Jefferson County, in which most of the water for public supply is purchased from purveyors outside the county, has a low county withdrawal rate and therefore has a low per capita rate. If no survey for a county was returned, a coefficient of 120 gal/d, which the CDWR updated in 2000, was used to estimate a groundwater or surface-water withdrawal. These per capita use rates also include public water use such as firefighting and municipal park irrigation, as well as losses due to system leakage.

The total quantity of water withdrawn for public-supply use in 2005 was estimated to be 864.17 Mgal/d (table 5), and the number of people served in Colorado was estimated to be 4.367 million or about 94 percent of the total population in the State. Counties with the largest total public-supply withdrawals (greater than 50 Mgal/d) were Denver, El Paso, Pueblo, Arapahoe, Larimer, and Adams (fig. 7). The majority of the public-supply drinking water for Coloradans came from a

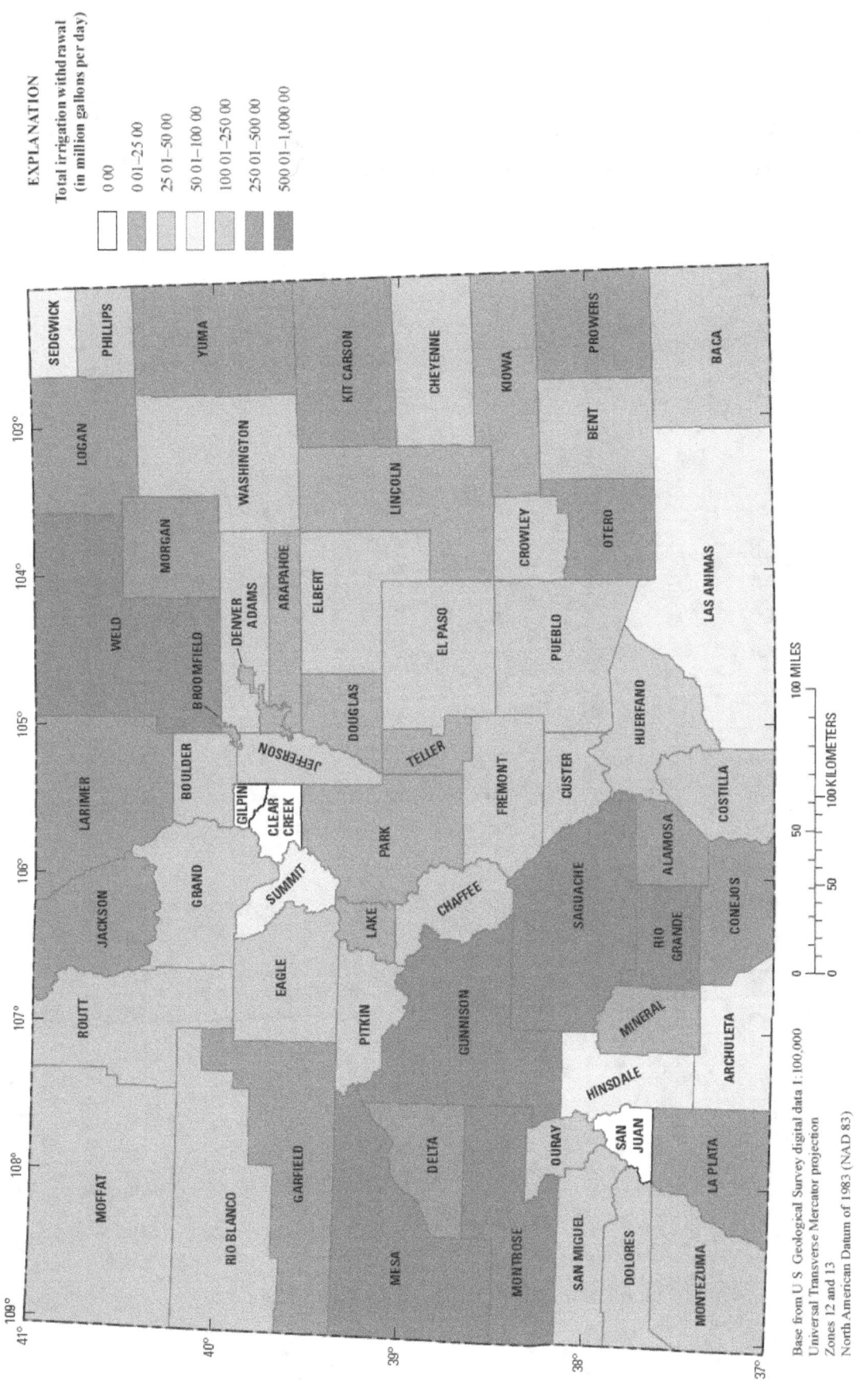

EXPLANATION

Total irrigation withdrawal
(in million gallons per day)

0 00
0 01–25 00
25 01–50 00
50 01–100 00
100 01–250 00
250 01–500 00
500 01–1,000 00

Base from U S Geological Survey digital data 1:100,000
Universal Transverse Mercator projection
Zones 12 and 13
North American Datum of 1983 (NAD 83)

Figure 6.   Estimated total irrigation (crop and golf course) water withdrawals by Colorado county, 2005.

Table 5.   Estimated public-supply water withdrawals and deliveries in Colorado by county, 2005.

[Mgal/d, million gallons per day; gal/d, gallons per day; per capita use based on either total public supply withdrawals or from public supply deliveries for domestic use]

County (fig. 2)	Population served (thousands)		Water withdrawals (Mgal/d)		Water deliveries for domestic use (Mgal/d)	Per capita use (gal/d)	
	Groundwater	Surface water	Groundwater	Surface water		Total public withdrawals	Domestic use
Adams	57.32	341.81	12.24	38.83	32.99	128	83
Alamosa	11.38	.00	2.00	0.00	1.54	176	135
Arapahoe	32.19	491.88	7.01	68.67	53.55	144	102
Archuleta	1.47	5.82	.07	.70	.74	106	102
Baca	2.89	.00	.75	.00	.24	260	83
Bent	4.26	.00	1.13	.00	.43	265	101
Boulder	2.38	275.86	.22	45.40	32.27	164	116
Broomfield	0.00	37.09	0.00	4.45	3.16	120	85
Chaffee	4.64	9.24	.58	1.11	1.41	122	102
Cheyenne	1.32	.00	.42	.00	.38	319	288
Clear Creek	1.29	5.20	.91	.39	.62	200	95
Conejos	4.85	.00	.87	.00	.76	179	157
Costilla	2.55	.00	.43	.00	.36	169	141
Crowley	4.50	.00	.79	.00	.35	176	78
Custer	1.09	.00	.12	.00	.12	110	110
Delta	5.92	16.01	.93	4.96	5.29	269	241
Denver	0.00	557.92	0.00	228.53	93.67	410	168
Dolores	0.00	1.20	0.00	.32	.23	267	192
Douglas	150.13	88.39	15.34	14.82	21.08	126	88
Eagle	20.45	27.00	4.02	5.17	6.53	194	138
Elbert	8.01	.00	1.05	.00	.91	131	114
El Paso	172.52	375.22	14.94	101.72	99.84	213	182
Fremont	.43	41.97	.05	7.55	3.02	179	71
Garfield	9.17	31.88	1.35	13.27	5.39	356	131
Gilpin	.10	3.58	.07	.44	.32	139	87
Grand	5.96	6.73	1.37	1.02	1.73	188	136
Gunnison	10.23	3.61	1.83	1.00	1.15	204	83
Hinsdale	.60	.00	.51	.00	.23	850	383
Huerfano	.88	6.52	.06	.79	.72	115	97
Jackson	.42	.38	.08	.10	.15	225	188
Jefferson	5.60	439.81	.82	8.81	29.56	22	66
Kiowa	1.01	.00	.14	.00	.11	138	109
Kit Carson	5.85	.00	1.51	.00	1.37	258	234

Table 5. Estimated public-supply water withdrawals and deliveries in Colorado by county, 2005.—Continued

[Mgal/d, million gallons per day; gal/d, gallons per day; per capita use based on either total public supply withdrawals or from public supply deliveries for domestic use]

County (fig. 2)	Population served (thousands)		Water withdrawals (Mgal/d)		Water deliveries for domestic use (Mgal/d)	Per capita use (gal/d)	
	Groundwater	Surface water	Groundwater	Surface water		Total public withdrawals	Domestic use
Lake	1.78	4.50	0.17	0.96	1.07	180	170
La Plata	9.08	34.09	.90	4.32	3.91	121	91
Larimer	1.36	268.33	.18	56.55	35.11	210	130
Las Animas	.99	10.52	.20	2.20	2.37	208	206
Lincoln	4.91	.00	.81	.00	.71	165	145
Logan	15.57	.00	2.54	.00	1.30	163	84
Mesa	1.64	125.37	.33	14.25	8.81	115	69
Mineral	.47	.00	.27	.00	.19	572	403
Moffat	.35	9.30	.06	1.54	1.14	166	118
Montezuma	.30	24.02	.03	2.56	2.40	107	99
Montrose	.60	34.87	.07	8.80	6.37	250	180
Morgan	14.58	12.00	3.38	2.78	5.23	232	197
Otero	14.56	4.29	4.34	.73	1.60	269	85
Ouray	2.88	.00	.35	.14	.35	170	121
Park	1.54	1.10	.26	.08	.29	129	110
Phillips	3.27	.00	1.66	.00	1.25	507	382
Pitkin	2.08	12.71	.51	3.87	2.73	296	185
Prowers	10.29	.00	1.80	.00	1.34	175	130
Pueblo	.46	148.75	.52	83.40	19.58	562	131
Rio Blanco	2.24	2.30	.60	.62	1.12	269	247
Rio Grande	7.03	.00	1.40	.00	1.11	199	158
Routt	2.14	14.93	.55	4.00	3.15	267	185
Saguache	3.22	.86	.64	.14	.62	191	152
San Juan	.00	.41	.00	.06	.05	146	122
San Miguel	.53	5.12	.06	.69	.51	133	90
Sedgwick	1.98	.00	.63	.00	.53	318	267
Summit	15.44	7.85	3.55	2.51	5.01	260	215
Teller	11.12	8.34	.82	.50	1.16	68	60
Washington	2.53	.00	.69	.00	0.33	273	130
Weld	8.66	192.72	.86	23.56	18.59	121	92
Yuma	6.06	.00	2.07	.00	1.36	341	224
Total	677.07	3,689.50	101.86	762.31	529.51	198[1]	121[1]

[1] Average per capita.

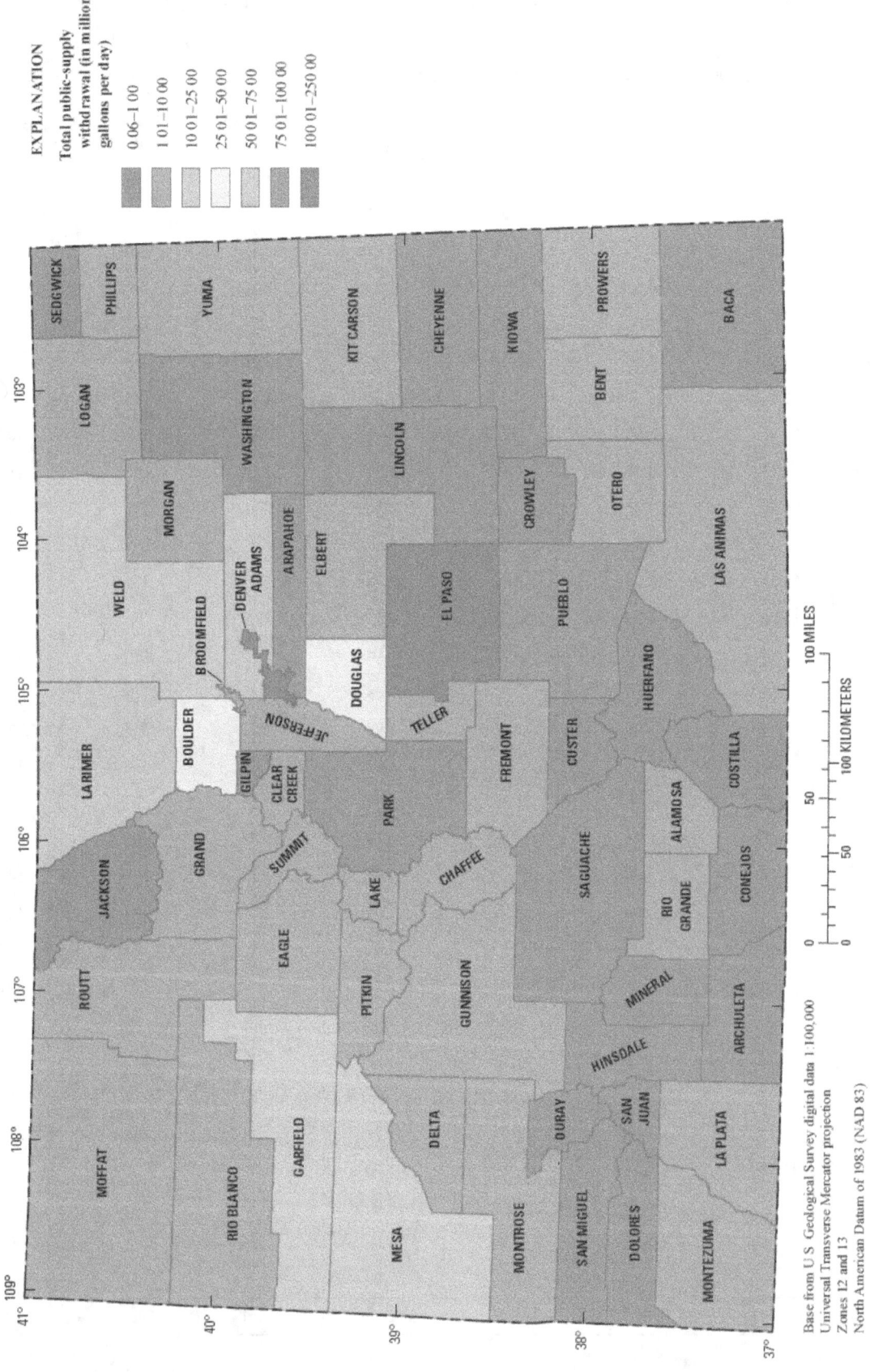

EXPLANATION

Total public-supply
withdrawal (in million
gallons per day)

0 06–1 00
1 01–10 00
10 01–25 00
25 01–50 00
50 01–75 00
75 01–100 00
100 01–250 00

Base from U S Geological Survey digital data 1 100,000
Universal Transverse Mercator projection
Zones 12 and 13
North American Datum of 1983 (NAD 83)

Figure 7.   Estimated total public-supply water withdrawals by Colorado county, 2005.

surface-water source (88.2 percent), and the counties with the largest surface-water withdrawals (greater than 50 Mgal/d) were Denver, El Paso, Pueblo, Arapahoe, and Larimer. The remaining 11.8 percent of public-supply water came from groundwater sources, and the counties with the greatest groundwater withdrawals were Douglas, El Paso, and Adams. A number of counties with small populations rely solely on groundwater for their public-water supplies (table 5), including counties in the Rio Grande Basin (fig. 1) and the eastern plains of Colorado.

Public-supply deliveries for domestic use totaled an estimated 529.51 Mgal/d, which is equivalent to an average per capita use of 121 gal/d. Per capita coefficients for deliveries for domestic use ranged from 60 gal/d (Teller County) to 403 gal/d (Mineral County) (table 5). The low estimated per capita coefficient for mountainous Teller County is attributed to a combination of higher precipitation in relation to other counties that are in the foothills of the Rocky Mountains and because many homeowners leave their yards in a more natural state, requiring little supplemental irrigation (Jim Schultz, Utilities Director, City of Woodland Park, oral commun., 2008). In Mineral County, the large per capita water use is attributed to losses through outdated water lines as well as the general practice of some homeowners bleeding water lines in the winter (allowing a slow steady stream of water to run through faucets) to prevent pipes from freezing. The town of Creede in Mineral County is in the process of upgrading the water infrastructure (Clyde Dooley, Creede City Manager, oral commun., 2008).

Self-Supplied Domestic

Water use for domestic purposes includes inside household purposes such as washing clothes, cleaning dishes, drinking, food preparation, bathing, and flushing toilets; outside uses are predominantly for watering lawns and gardens. The population of Colorado that has self-supplied domestic water was determined by subtracting the number of people served by public-supply systems in a county from the total county population as reported by the U.S. Census Bureau (2006). This number was then multiplied by a per capita use coefficient for the county, derived from the county public-supply domestic deliveries (table 6) to estimate self-supplied domestic-water withdrawals.

In Colorado, all self-supplied domestic-water use is from a groundwater source; well withdrawals for 2005 totaled 34.43 Mgal/d, serving an estimated population of 298,610. The average estimated domestic per capita water use was 115 gal/d. Counties with the largest withdrawals (greater than 1 Mgal/d) were Jefferson, El Paso, Weld, Delta, Elbert, Park, and Garfield (table 6; fig. 8). Consumptive use for self-supplied domestic water use was assumed to be 10 percent of withdrawals (Don West, Water Resources Engineer, Colorado Division of Water Resources, written commun., 2008), and is similar to the ratio used by engineers in designing septic systems. Thus, the total consumptive use for self-supplied domestic withdrawals was estimated as 3.44 Mgal/d.

Self-Supplied Industrial

Industrial water is used primarily in the manufacturing process, including facilities that produce food, steel, machinery, chemical and allied products, and paper and pulp mills. This also includes printing and publishing facilities and petroleum refining. Water used in the process of power generation, and mineral mining or extraction of crude petroleum or gasses is not included in this water-use category. Estimates of withdrawals for self-supplied industrial-water use were taken directly from the 2005 CDWR database, and are assumed to be strictly the self-supplied users. The CDWR provided both groundwater and surface-water withdrawals by county, and no other source water (such as reclaimed water) was provided in the dataset.

In 2005, a total of 7,342 industries were located in Colorado, according to the Manufacturers' News, Inc. (2005), of which the principal employing industry groups in the State (in decreasing order of approximate number of employees) were communications equipment, newspapers, air/spacecraft manufacturers, prepackaged computer software, and commercial printers. Self-supplied industrial-water withdrawals in Colorado totaled an estimated 142.44 Mgal/d and ranged from little or no withdrawals in many counties to greater than 30 Mgal/d in Pueblo and Jefferson Counties (fig. 9, table 7). Surface water supplied 97.5 percent (138.83 Mgal/d) of the water to Colorado industries.

Livestock

Livestock water use pertains to the commercial production of meat, milk, poultry, eggs, and wool. Livestock water use was estimated according to methods described by Lovelace (2009a). These estimates were based on the 2002 Agricultural Census (U.S. Department of Agriculture, 2002) inventory of animals in each county in Colorado, and a daily per head consumption rate for the various types of livestock (table 8). Livestock water-use estimates are shown in table 9. Proportions of groundwater and surface-water sources in each county were based on the 1985 compilation (Litke and Appel, 1989) and updated for Weld County based on CDWR information (table 9).

Water use for livestock in 2005 was estimated to be 33.06 Mgal/d, which is less than 1 percent of the total water use in Colorado. Five counties in northeastern Colorado (Weld, Yuma, Morgan, Logan, and Kit Carson) had 53.4 percent of the State's estimated 2.7 million bovine (both dairy and beef), of which 20.6 percent were in Weld County alone (U.S. Department of Agriculture, 2002). Prowers County, in the Arkansas River Basin (1102), was the only other county with greater than 100,000 head of cattle, and similar to the other counties with large numbers of cattle, is

Table 6.   Estimated self-supplied domestic-water withdrawals in Colorado by county, 2005.

[Mgal/d, million gallons per day; gal/d, gallons per day]

County (fig. 2)	Self-supplied population (thousands)	Groundwater withdrawals (Mgal/d)	Per capita use (gal/d)
Adams	0.29	0.02	68
Alamosa	3.90	.53	136
Arapahoe	5.02	.51	102
Archuleta	4.60	.47	102
Baca	1.18	.10	85
Bent	1.30	.13	100
Boulder	2.20	.25	114
Broomfield	6.39	.54	85
Chaffee	3.09	.31	100
Cheyenne	.64	.18	283
Clear Creek	2.70	.26	96
Conejos	3.66	.57	156
Costilla	.88	.12	137
Crowley	.90	.07	78
Custer	2.77	.31	112
Delta	8.02	1.93	241
Denver	.00	.00	0
Dolores	.63	.12	191
Douglas	10.90	.96	88
Eagle	.07	.01	139
Elbert	14.78	1.68	114
El Paso	17.84	3.25	182
Fremont	5.37	.38	71
Garfield	8.76	1.15	131
Gilpin	1.25	.11	88
Grand	.52	.07	135
Gunnison	.39	.03	78
Hinsdale	.17	.06	364
Huerfano	.38	.04	106
Jackson	.65	.12	185
Jefferson	81.40	5.71	70
Kiowa	.41	.04	98
Kit Carson	1.79	.42	234

Table 6. Estimated self-supplied domestic-water withdrawals in Colorado by county, 2005.—Continued

[Mgal/d, million gallons per day; gal/d, gallons per day]

County (fig. 2)	Self-supplied population (thousands)	Groundwater withdrawals (Mgal/d)	Per capita use (gal/d)
Lake	1.46	0.25	172
La Plata	4.28	.39	91
Larimer	2.24	.29	129
Las Animas	3.93	.81	206
Lincoln	.71	.10	141
Logan	5.15	.43	83
Mesa	2.86	.20	70
Mineral	.46	.18	391
Moffat	3.77	.44	117
Montezuma	.46	.05	109
Montrose	2.01	.36	179
Morgan	1.41	.28	198
Otero	.65	.05	77
Ouray	1.38	.17	124
Park	14.31	1.57	110
Phillips	1.31	.50	381
Pitkin	.12	.02	163
Prowers	3.60	.47	131
Pueblo	2.11	.57	270
Rio Blanco	1.43	.35	245
Rio Grande	5.20	.82	158
Routt	4.24	.78	184
Saguache	2.95	.45	153
San Juan	.17	.02	120
San Miguel	1.56	.14	90
Sedgwick	.55	.15	274
Summit	1.60	.34	213
Teller	2.46	.15	61
Washington	2.10	.28	133
Weld	27.56	2.54	92
Yuma	3.72	.83	223
Total	298.61	34.43	115[1]

[1] Average per capita.

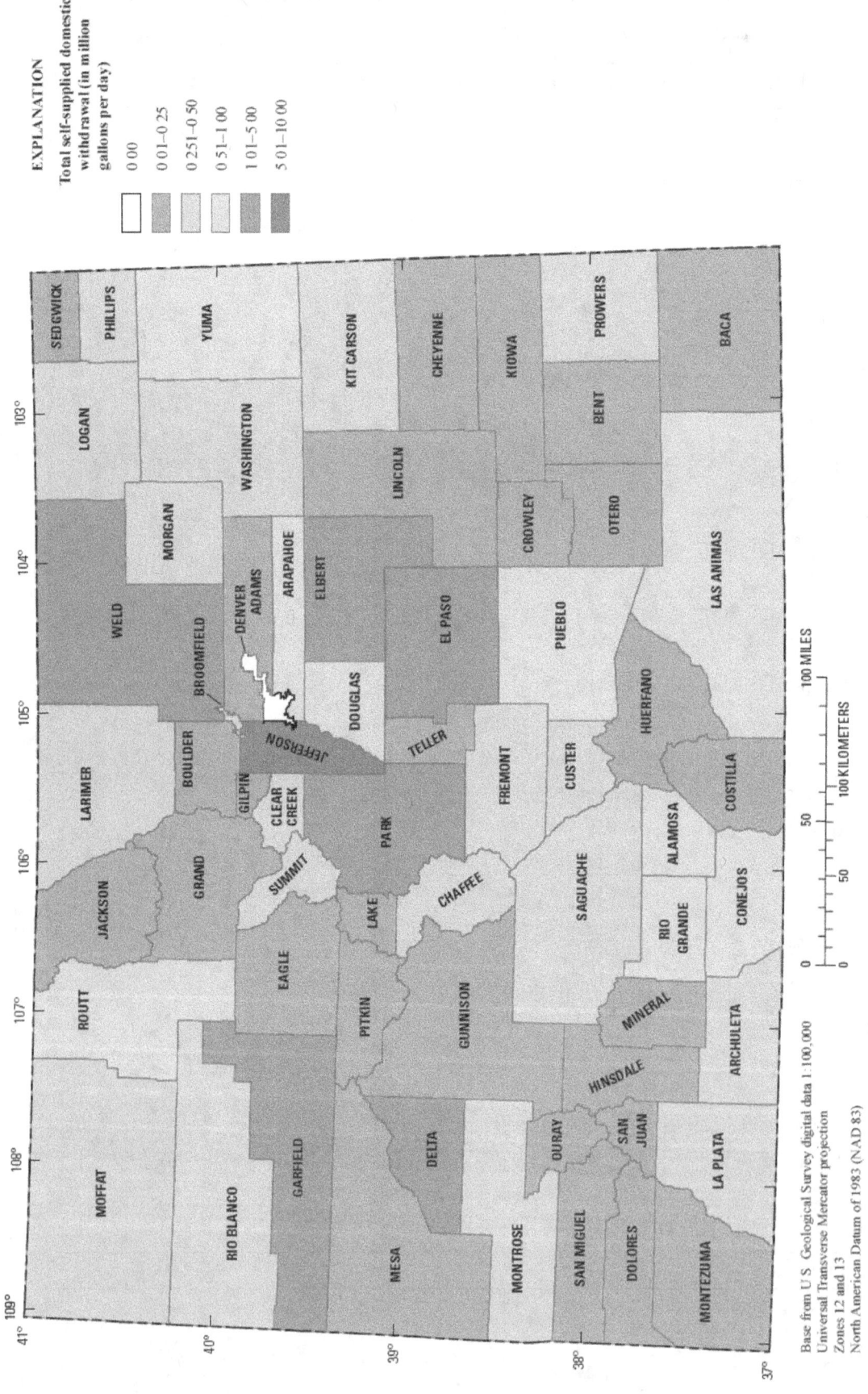

Figure 8.   Estimated total self-supplied domestic-water withdrawals by Colorado county, 2005.

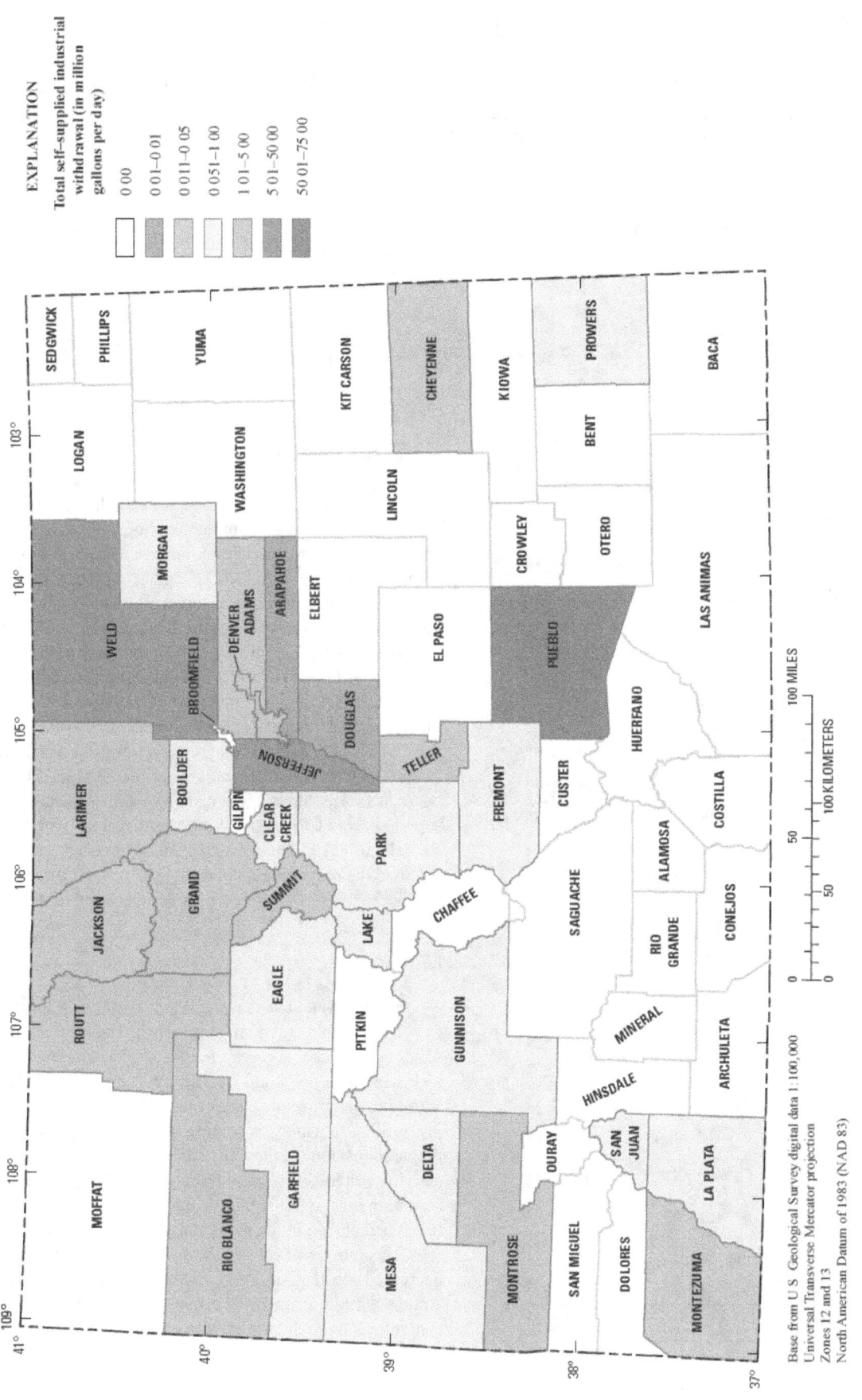

Figure 9.   Estimated total self-supplied industrial-water withdrawals by Colorado county, 2005.

Table 7. Estimated self-supplied industrial-water withdrawals in Colorado by county, 2005.

[Counties with no withdrawal are not listed; Mgal/d, million gallons per day]

County (fig. 2)	Withdrawals by source, in Mgal/d	
	Groundwater	Surface water
Adams	0.71	1.73
Arapahoe	.01	.00
Boulder	.00	.41
Cheyenne	.00	.02
Clear Creek	.00	.07
Delta	.00	.23
Denver	.00	4.21
Douglas	.01	.00
Eagle	.00	.26
Fremont	.00	.49
Garfield	.00	.50
Grand	.00	1.39
Gunnison	.00	.67
Jackson	.00	.02
Jefferson	.15	39.23
Lake	.00	.14
La Plata	.00	.44
Larimer	.00	3.36
Mesa	.00	.55
Montezuma	.00	.05
Montrose	.00	1.77
Morgan	.47	.44
Park	.00	.56
Prowers	.00	.25
Pueblo	.00	72.32
Rio Blanco	.00	2.33
Routt	.00	3.01
San Juan	.00	.18
Summit	.00	.02
Teller	.00	1.21
Weld	2.26	2.97
Total	3.61	138.83

Table 8. Livestock water requirements.

Animal	Gallons per day per head[1]
Horses	12
Beef cattle	10
Dairy cattle	10
Hogs	3
Sheep	1
Goats	2
Chickens	.06

[1] Lovelace (2009a).

located east of the Continental Divide (fig. 2). Swine (about 437,490 head) also are primarily produced in the eastern part of the State, where Yuma (81 percent) and Logan (9.9 percent) Counties had the largest numbers of hogs. Sheep have been mostly raised in the western part of the State (Litke and Appel, 1989), and 36 percent of the sheep were in Moffat, Rio Blanco, and Delta Counties. However, Weld County, east of the Continental Divide, reported 36 percent (133,857 head) of Colorado's sheep in 2002. Weld County also had the greatest percentage of chickens (98.7 percent), goats (14.8 percent), and equine (8.5 percent) of the State's total populations for those livestock reported and led counties in livestock water use (7.12 Mgal/d, combined groundwater and surface water) (table 9). Other counties with greater than 2 Mgal/d livestock water use were Yuma, Morgan, and Logan. Groundwater supplied about 67 percent of the total livestock withdrawals for animals (22.11 Mgal/d), whereas surface-water sources supplied the remaining 33 percent (10.95 Mgal/d). All water for livestock use was assumed to be consumptively used.

Mining

Mining water use is water that is withdrawn for the extraction of fuel and nonfuel minerals. These minerals are solids such as coal and ores, liquids such as crude petroleum, and gases such as natural gas and coal-bed methane. The water is used in the process of quarrying, oil and gas well dewatering, milling (crushing, screening, and washing), and other preparations done at the mine site or as part of the mining activity. Water used as part of the processing of raw materials (smelting ores, refining petroleum, and slurry pipeline operations) is included in the industrial water-use category.

The number of active hard-rock mines in Colorado has decreased substantially from 150 mines in 1985 (Litke and Appel, 1989) to 20 in 2005. Of these 20 active mines, 13 were coal mines, 8 of which were underground and 5 were surface

Table 9.   Estimated livestock water withdrawals in Colorado by county, 2005.

[Counties with no withdrawals are not listed; Mgal/d, million gallons per day]

County (fig. 2)	Groundwater withdrawals (Mgal/d)	Surface-water withdrawals (Mgal/d)	Total withdrawals (Mgal/d)
Adams	0.17	0.05	0.22
Alamosa	.11	.02	.13
Arapahoe	.11	.01	.12
Archuleta	.02	.07	.09
Baca	.70	.04	.74
Bent	.40	.33	.73
Boulder	.04	.14	.18
Chaffee	.01	.07	.08
Cheyenne	.18	.03	.21
Conejos	.08	.21	.29
Costilla	.05	.04	.09
Crowley	.24	.09	.33
Custer	.02	.04	.06
Delta	.17	.23	.40
Dolores	.01	.02	.03
Douglas	.05	.07	.12
Eagle	.02	.06	.08
Elbert	.36	.11	.47
El Paso	.23	.12	.35
Fremont	.06	.12	.18
Garfield	.11	.16	.27
Grand	.04	.12	.16
Gunnison	.02	.15	.17
Hinsdale	.00	.02	.02
Huerfano	.02	.10	.12
Jackson	.00	.25	.25
Jefferson	.01	.05	.06
Kiowa	.16	.06	.22
Kit Carson	1.19	.28	1.47
Lake	.00	.00	.00
La Plata	.06	.20	.26
Larimer	.20	.72	.92

Table 9.   Estimated livestock water withdrawals in Colorado by county, 2005.—Continued

[Counties with no withdrawals are not listed; Mgal/d, million gallons per day]

County (fig. 2)	Groundwater withdrawals (Mgal/d)	Surface-water withdrawals (Mgal/d)	Total withdrawals (Mgal/d)
Las Animas	0.15	0.29	0.44
Lincoln	.37	.11	.48
Logan	1.48	.80	2.28
Mesa	.09	.48	.57
Mineral	.00	.01	.01
Moffat	.20	.25	.45
Montezuma	.03	.20	.23
Montrose	.18	.44	.62
Morgan	1.88	1.08	2.96
Otero	.35	.35	.70
Ouray	.01	.07	.08
Park	.00	.10	.10
Phillips	.48	.05	.53
Pitkin	.00	.02	.02
Prowers	.32	.90	1.22
Pueblo	.17	.22	.39
Rio Blanco	.06	.22	.28
Rio Grande	.07	.08	.15
Routt	.07	.27	.34
Saguache	.09	.20	.29
San Miguel	.04	.05	.09
Sedgwick	.28	.10	.38
Summit	.01	.02	.03
Teller	.00	.03	.03
Washington	.57	.10	.67
Weld	7.07	.05	7.12
Yuma	3.30	.48	3.78
Total	22.11	10.95	33.06

mines. These mines produced 37.8 million tons of coal, and employed a maximum of 2,314 miners in Delta, Moffat, Rio Blanco, Gunnison, Routt, Montrose, La Plata, and Garfield Counties (Colorado Division of Reclamation Mining and Safety, 2008). The remaining 7 active hard-rock mines in Colorado in 2005 consisted of 4 uranium/vanadium, 1 gold, 1 gold/silver, and 1 molybdenum mine (Cappa and others, 2006). All the uranium/vanadium (vanadium is a coproduct of the uranium production) mines were located in Montrose County, where a total of 127.8 tons of uranium and 687.3 tons of vanadium were produced. Gold production totaled 11.1 tons: 10.3 tons from a surface mine in Teller County and 0.8 ton from an underground mine in Hinsdale County. Silver is a coproduct of gold mining from the surface mine in Teller County; a total of 5.3 tons of silver was produced in 2005. A single underground mine in Clear Creek County produced 16,101 tons of molybdenum.

In 2005, 47 million tons of sand, gravel, and construction aggregate were produced from about 1,150 operations located in nearly every county in Colorado. Source water for the sand and gravel operations was nearly 100-percent groundwater with each mine using approximately 0.004 Mgal/d (David L. Nettles, Assistant Division 1 Engineer, Colorado Division of Water Resources, written commun., 2008). Water in sand and gravel operations is recycled through settling ponds and reused until its complete consumption in the aggregate washing process. Evaporation from the settling ponds also is included in the 0.004 Mgal/d estimate. Freshwater withdrawals for coal, hard-rock, and construction materials mining were estimated to be 5.20 Mgal/d from groundwater and 1.24 Mgal/d from surface water (table 10). Total water use for coal mining (both ground and fresh/saline surface water) was estimated to be 2.66 Mgal/d, and hard-rock mines and the sand/gravel quarries used about 0.01 and 4.17 Mgal/d of groundwater, respectively.

Records of water produced at oil and gas fields in Colorado during 2005 were obtained from the Colorado Oil and Gas Conservation Commission (2007). The data included county, volume of water produced, and a water disposal code. The following assumptions were used in determining water use based on work by Lovelace (2009b): (1) all water coded as "I" was injected for secondary oil or gas recovery or some related beneficial use and was considered a groundwater withdrawal; (2) all other water (central disposal, commercial disposal, pit, surface discharge, and undefined) was considered produced water that was disposed of as waste, with no beneficial use, and was not included as a withdrawal; and (3) all injected water was assumed to be saline groundwater. An estimated 14.59 Mgal/d of saline water was withdrawn

and reinjected in 2005 and was considered by the USGS as a beneficial use. The counties with the largest amount of oil and gas mining water withdrawals were Rio Blanco, Las Animas, and Moffat, and the same counties also had the largest total mining water withdrawals (fig. 10, table 10).

Thermoelectric

Thermoelectric-power water use is subdivided by fuel type, and data were compiled by source-water type, water-supply method, water disposition type, and power generated. In this report, all water withdrawals for thermoelectric power generation are self-supplied, and any water provided through public-supply systems is documented in the public-supply withdrawal category. Most of the data for this water-use category were compiled by the Energy Information Administration and provided by the NWUIP; however, water-use information is collected only for the large non-nuclear power generating plants, those with a capacity of 100 megawatts or greater. For powerplants with capacity between 10 and 99 megawatts, no cooling system (water-use) information is required, but power generation is reported. Powerplants with capacities between 10 and 99 megawatts were contacted for water-use information. All 24 thermoelectric plants in Colorado (fig. 11) are fossil-fuel plants, which are a variety of types, ranging from diesel generators that use very little water in the cooling process to five once-through plants where large volumes of water are passed through the cooling structures and returned to the natural system with nearly no water consumed. The 14 (mostly coal-fired) closed-loop plants recycle the same water through the cooling system until the water is essentially consumed, withdrawing much less water than the once-through plants.

Total water withdrawn for 2005 thermoelectric power generation was estimated to be 123.21 Mgal/d (table 11) of which surface-water sources accounted for 94.7 percent. Consumptive use was 43.44 Mgal/d, with an average consumption rate for the 14 closed-loop plants of 84 percent of the withdrawn water. Counties with the greatest total withdrawals were Mesa, Pueblo, and Fremont (table 11). A total of 38,174.40 gigawatt-hours of electricity were generated in 2005 by powerplants using water for cooling.

As an alternative to fossil-fuel electric generation (and using no water) in Colorado are wind turbine facilities and solar energy arrays. Currently (2005) Colorado has two wind farms, one each in Weld and Logan Counties, that combined produced 132.3 gigawatt-hours of power (Cappa and others, 2006). In 2005, no large-scale solar arrays were in operation.

Table 10.   Estimated mining water withdrawals in Colorado by county, 2005.

[Mgal/d, million gallons per day; counties with no withdrawal are not listed]

County (fig. 2)	Withdrawals (Mgal/d)			
	Groundwater (fresh)	Groundwater (saline)	Surface water (fresh)	Surface water (saline)
Adams	0.14	0.03	0.00	0.00
Alamosa	.01	.00	.00	.00
Arapahoe	.02	.01	.00	.00
Archuleta	.07	.03	.00	.00
Baca	.04	.29	.00	.00
Bent	.06	.00	.00	.00
Boulder	.05	.00	.00	.00
Chaffee	.05	.00	.00	.00
Cheyenne	.06	.30	.00	.00
Clear Creek	.01	.00	.00	.00
Conejos	.03	.00	.00	.00
Costilla	.03	.00	.00	.00
Crowely	.02	.00	.00	.00
Custer	.03	.00	.00	.00
Delta	.39	.00	.23	.00
Dolores	.01	.02	.00	.00
Douglas	.03	.00	.00	.00
Eagle	.04	.00	.00	.00
Elbert	.08	.03	.00	.00
El Paso	.05	.00	.00	.00
Fremont	.12	.00	.00	.00
Garfield	.07	.00	.00	.00
Grand	.06	.00	.00	.00
Gunnison	.29	.00	.00	.00
Hinsdale	.01	.00	.00	.00
Huerfano	.09	.00	.00	.00
Jackson	.04	.15	.00	.00
Jefferson	.03	.00	.00	.00
Kiowa	.03	.04	.00	.00
Kit Carson	.11	.02	.00	.00
Lake	.15	.00	.00	.00

Table 10. Estimated mining water withdrawals in Colorado by county, 2005.—Continued

[Mgal/d, million gallons per day; counties with no withdrawal are not listed]

County (fig. 2)	Withdrawals (Mgal/d)			
	Groundwater (fresh)	Groundwater (saline)	Surface water (fresh)	Surface water (saline)
La Plata	0.03	0.30	0.00	0.00
Larimer	.18	.33	.00	.00
Las Animas	.09	1.46	.00	.00
Lincoln	.11	.01	.00	.00
Logan	.13	.43	.00	.00
Mesa	.21	.00	.00	.00
Mineral	.01	.00	.00	.00
Moffat	.16	.49	.08	.39
Montezuma	.04	.02	.00	.00
Montrose	.19	.00	.43	.00
Morgan	.10	.20	.00	.00
Otero	.06	.00	.00	.00
Ouray	.02	.00	.00	.00
Park	.07	.00	.00	.00
Phillips	.05	.02	.00	.00
Pitkin	.01	.00	.00	.00
Prowers	.11	.00	.00	.00
Pueblo	.12	.00	.00	.00
Rio Blanco	.10	9.46	.36	.00
Rio Grande	.06	.00	.00	.00
Routt	.45	.00	.14	.00
Saguache	.06	.00	.00	.00
San Juan	.01	.00	.00	.00
San Miguel	.04	.00	.00	.00
Sedgwick	.02	.00	.00	.00
Summit	.01	.00	.00	.00
Teller	.04	.00	.00	.00
Washington	.08	.51	.00	.00
Weld	.35	.33	.00	.00
Yuma	.07	.11	.00	.00
Total	5.20	14.59	1.24	0.39

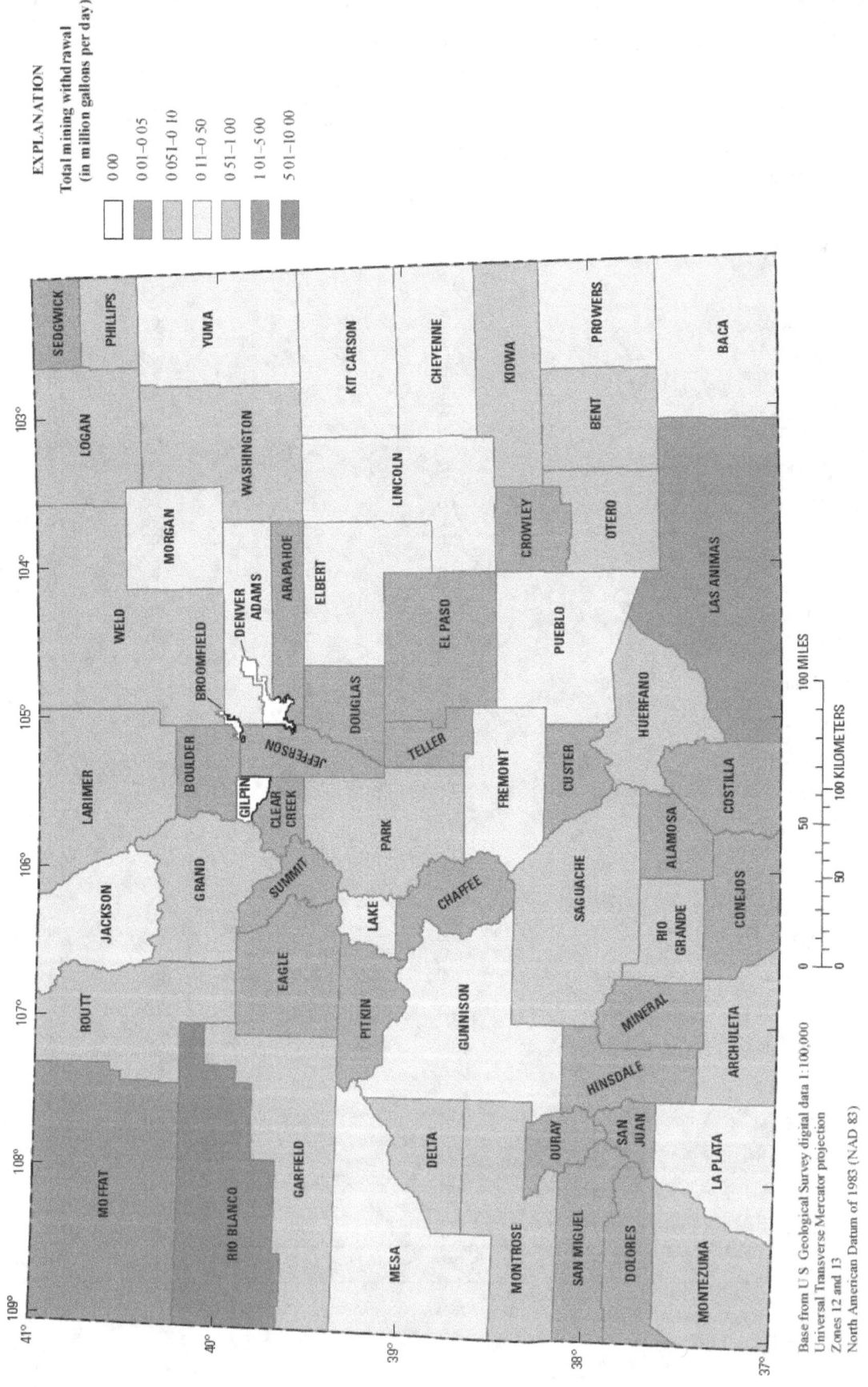

Figure 10.   Estimated total mining water withdrawals by Colorado county, 2005.

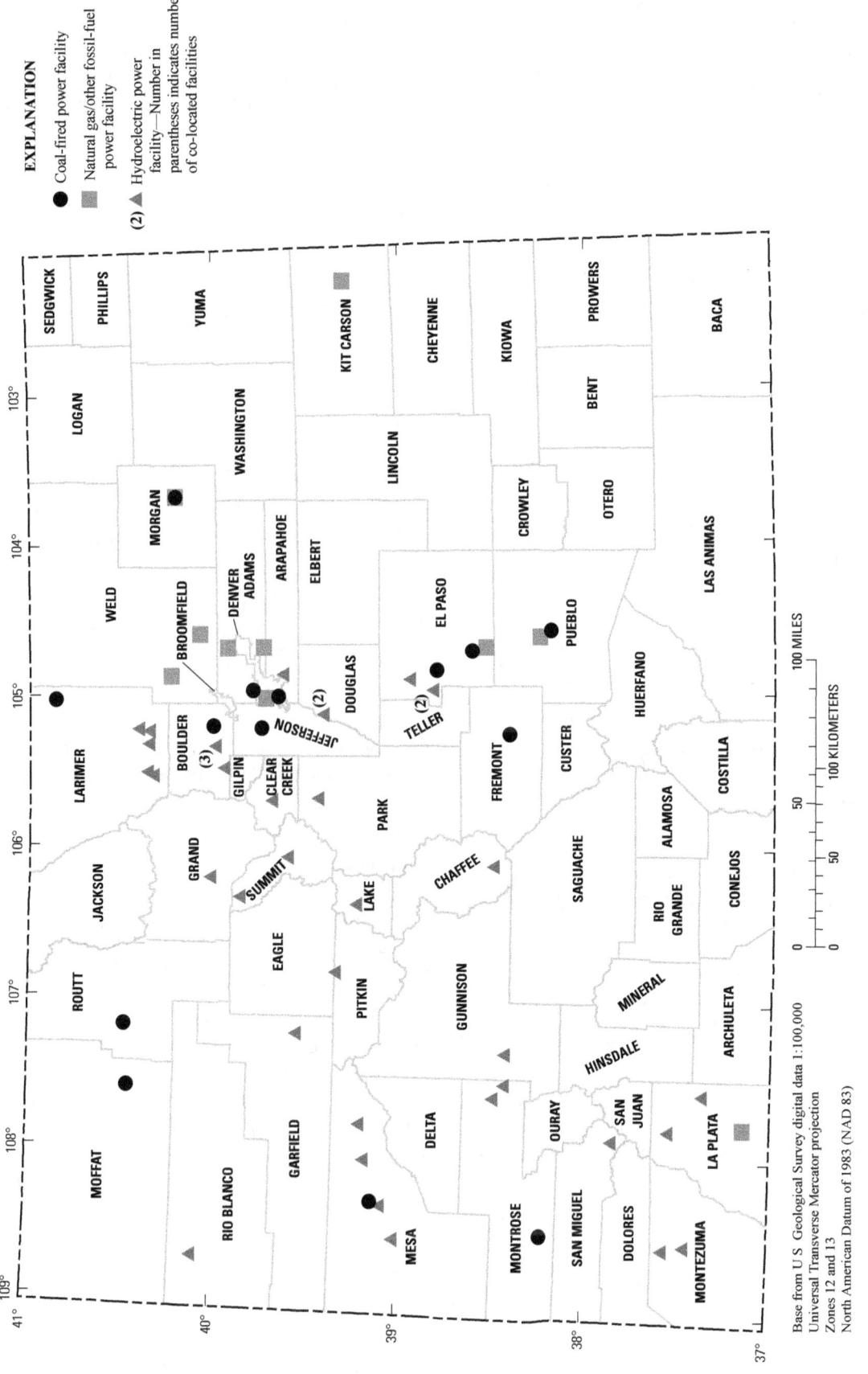

Figure 11.   Locations of coal, natural gas and other fossil-fuel (water cooled), and hydroelectric power generating facilities in Colorado, 2005.

Base from U S Geological Survey digital data 1:100,000
Universal Transverse Mercator projection
Zones 12 and 13
North American Datum of 1983 (NAD 83)

Table 11.   Water withdrawals and consumption for thermoelectric power generation in Colorado by county, 2005.

[Counties with no withdrawal are not listed; Mgal/d, million gallons per day; GWh, gigawatt-hours]

County (fig. 2)	Withdrawals (Mgal/d)			Consumption (Mgal/d)	Power generated (GWh)
	Groundwater	Surface water	Total		
Adams	0.01	9.24	9.25	6.98	5,257.02
Boulder	.00	5.82	5.82	3.30	1,500.72
Denver	.00	2.26	2.26	1.55	898.13
El Paso	2.54	.00	2.54	2.52	1,759.64
Fremont	.00	15.48	15.48	.00	290.58
Jefferson	.00	.03	.03	.00	298.20
Kit Carson	.01	.00	.01	.00	1.82
Mesa	.00	43.85	43.85	.00	3,972.10
Moffat	.00	12.81	12.81	12.81	10,116.20
Montrose	.00	1.68	1.68	1.42	736.96
Morgan	3.94	.00	3.94	3.94	3,022.42
Pueblo	.00	18.88	18.88	6.01	4,299.26
Routt	.00	2.52	2.52	2.52	3,146.35
Weld	.00	4.14	4.14	2.39	2,831.25
Total	6.50	116.71	123.21	43.44	38,174.40

Instream Hydroelectric Power Generation

Water used for the generation of hydroelectric power is considered an instream use, is nonconsumptive, and is withdrawn for only short times and distances. Information for this water use is included in this report because hydroelectric plants have rights to water that is not available for upstream consumption. Data for the amount of water withdrawn for power generation is considered very good because all but 2 of the 37 plants located in Colorado responded with information. Power generation information was provided by the U.S. Department of Energy (2006). The locations of the hydroelectric plants are shown in figure 11. Total hydroelectric water use in 2005 was 5,253.6 Mgal/d, and produced 1,599.45 gigawatt-hours of electricity (table 12). Colorado ranks 21st in the Nation for the amount of renewable hydroelectric energy production (National Priorities Project Database, 2001), and in 2005, hydroelectric power accounted for 5 percent of the total Colorado electric output (Cappa and others, 2006).

Other Water Uses

A few water uses were not included in this study. Water use by fish hatcheries (aquaculture), reservoir evaporation (except in the mining category), and water augmentation plans were not investigated. A few instream water uses such as water for aquatic habitat protection, recreational uses, and water-quality-maintenance uses also were not included. Undoubtedly, other water uses in Colorado have been overlooked, and some water uses are difficult to quantify, whereas others require a more expanded water-use-data classification structure.

Table 12. Instream water use for hydroelectric power generation in Colorado by county, 2005.

[Counties with no withdrawal are not listed; Mgal/d, million gallons per day; GWh, gigawatt-hours]

County (fig. 11)	Surface water (Mgal/d)	Power generated (GWh)	Number of operating facilities
Boulder	8.28	27.20	3
Chaffee	16.59	7.67	1
Clear Creek	52.66	3.36	1
Denver	110.00	14.56	2
Douglas	34.03	6.56	1
El Paso	45.46	72.17	3
Garfield	632.11	86.91	1
Grand	60.02	9.31	1
Gunnison	585.77	206.87	1
Jefferson	39.30	5.94	1
Lake	101.23	4.73	1
La Plata	381.23	48.57	2
Larimer	678.99	388.82	5
Mesa	223.48	68.73	4
Montezuma	339.54	154.83	2
Montrose	1,466.45	411.34	2
Park	39.66	11.20	1
Pitkin	194.58	15.82	1
Rio Blanco	53.87	11.61	1
San Miguel	23.23	7.74	1
Summit	167.12	35.51	2
Total	5,253.60	1,599.45	37

Water Withdrawals by Selected Aquifer

The Denver Basin aquifer, a system of sandstone, conglomerate, and shale aquifers that underlies about 7,000 mi^2 of the plains along the eastern front of the Rocky Mountains in Colorado, is composed of the following units, the Upper Dawson, Lower Dawson, Denver, Upper Arapahoe, Lower Arapahoe, and the Laramie-Fox Hills aquifers (fig. 12). A Quaternary alluvial aquifer overlies the Denver Basin system and is included in the water-use estimates. This aquifer system supplies water to rural and suburban residents as well as commercial establishments and some irrigation wells from Greeley to Colorado Springs and the greater Denver metropolitan area. The Denver Basin aquifer is not well connected to other major aquifers in the area and only a small portion (40,000 acre-ft) of the average 5 million acre-ft of precipitation is thought to recharge the Basin aquifers (U.S. Geological Survey, 2009). The Denver area has a long history of water level declines, and groundwater withdrawals have caused a decrease in the volume of groundwater in storage (U.S. Geological Survey, 2009). Because of the concern for the continuing availability of groundwater from the Denver Basin system, a groundwater model of the historical aquifer pumpage, as well as simulations of hypothetical future aquifer demands were built using MODFLOW (Paschke, 2010).

Fresh groundwater withdrawals were estimated for bedrock and overlying alluvial aquifers in the Denver Basin for crop irrigation, public supply, commercial/industrial, household-use only, and domestic/livestock water-use categories. Withdrawals were calculated for input into the USGS Denver Basin model (Paschke, 2010) for the period 1880 through 2004. In this report, only the information for the final year, 2004, is presented for the purpose of providing some compilation information on specific aquifer system withdrawals.

The primary data source for the calculated pumpage was based on the Well Permit database maintained by the CDWR. A total of 412,974 well records were transmitted from the CDWR, and after screening to eliminate wells lacking location, depth, or water-use information, a final dataset included 59,536 well records. The methodology for calculating pumpage for wells in the Denver Basin was to use the equations in the Senate Bill 96-074 groundwater model (Colorado Division of Water Resources, 1998). A full description of the approach and methods for calculating pumpage for wells in the Denver Basin are reported in Paschke (2010).

The greatest total withdrawals from any aquifer were from public-supply wells, and the least were from household-use-only wells (table 13). Douglas County had the greatest total withdrawals (183.98 Mgal/d), whereas Broomfield County had the smallest (3.09 Mgal/d). Of the seven Denver Basin aquifers, the Lower Arapahoe aquifer had the greatest total estimated withdrawals (287.11 Mgal/d), and Douglas County had the greatest public-supply withdrawal of any other county (95.29 Mgal/d) from this same aquifer. The Upper Dawson aquifer was the least used of the Denver

Basin aquifers, based on an estimated total withdrawal of 17.64 Mgal/d.

Comparison of the Colorado Statewide Water Supply Initiative Baseline Forecasted Water Demand for 2005 to Select 2005 Water-Use Estimates

As part of the Colorado Statewide Water Supply Initiative (SWSI) (Colorado Water Conservation Board, 2004), forecasts of future water demand were made on the basis of information such as population, climate, and 2000 water-use information. These baseline water demand forecasts were made for municipal, industrial, and select self-supplied (snow-making, power generation, and miscellaneous) water-use categories and did not include the effects of future water conservation. Forecasts for each year from 2000 through 2030 and for each Colorado county and river basin were calculated based on population projections and county gallon-per-capita water-use rates (Colorado Water Conservation Board, 2004). Categories compared between the SWSI baseline forecasted water demand and estimates in the USGS compilation were limited to county population, water use for municipal (public-supply)/industrial, and water use for self-supplied thermoelectric power generation. Public supply and industrial water use were separate categories in the USGS compilation; however, these estimates were combined to compare to the SWSI municipal/industrial baseline-forecasted values.

Population projections (in yearly increments from 2000 to 2030) used in the SWSI forecasts were obtained directly from the Colorado Department of Local Affairs (Colorado Water Conservation Board, 2004), whereas interim census year population estimates (U.S. Census Bureau, 2006) were used in the USGS compilation. Comparison of 2005 population estimates between the SWSI forecasts and the USGS 2005 compilation showed that 40 of the 64 counties had a difference between −5 and 5 percent, and 59 of the counties (92 percent) had a difference between −10 and 10 percent (table 14). Population estimates (based on 2005 interim values from the U.S. Census Bureau) used in the USGS compilation are less than the projections used in the SWSI forecast for the five counties where the population difference was greater than −10 percent. For all 64 counties, the population difference ranged from −11.89 to 10.87 percent with a median difference of −2.85 percent.

Five counties had a difference between −5 and 5 percent when comparing the combined municipal and industrial water-use categories between the SWSI baseline-forecasted water demand and the USGS compilation (table 14). In the same comparison, nine counties had a difference between −10 and 10 percent, and 38 counties had a difference between −50 and 50 percent. Three counties had a difference greater than or equal to 100 percent. Of the 64 Colorado counties, 49 (77 percent) had a municipal/industrial USGS water-use estimate that was lower than the SWSI water-demand

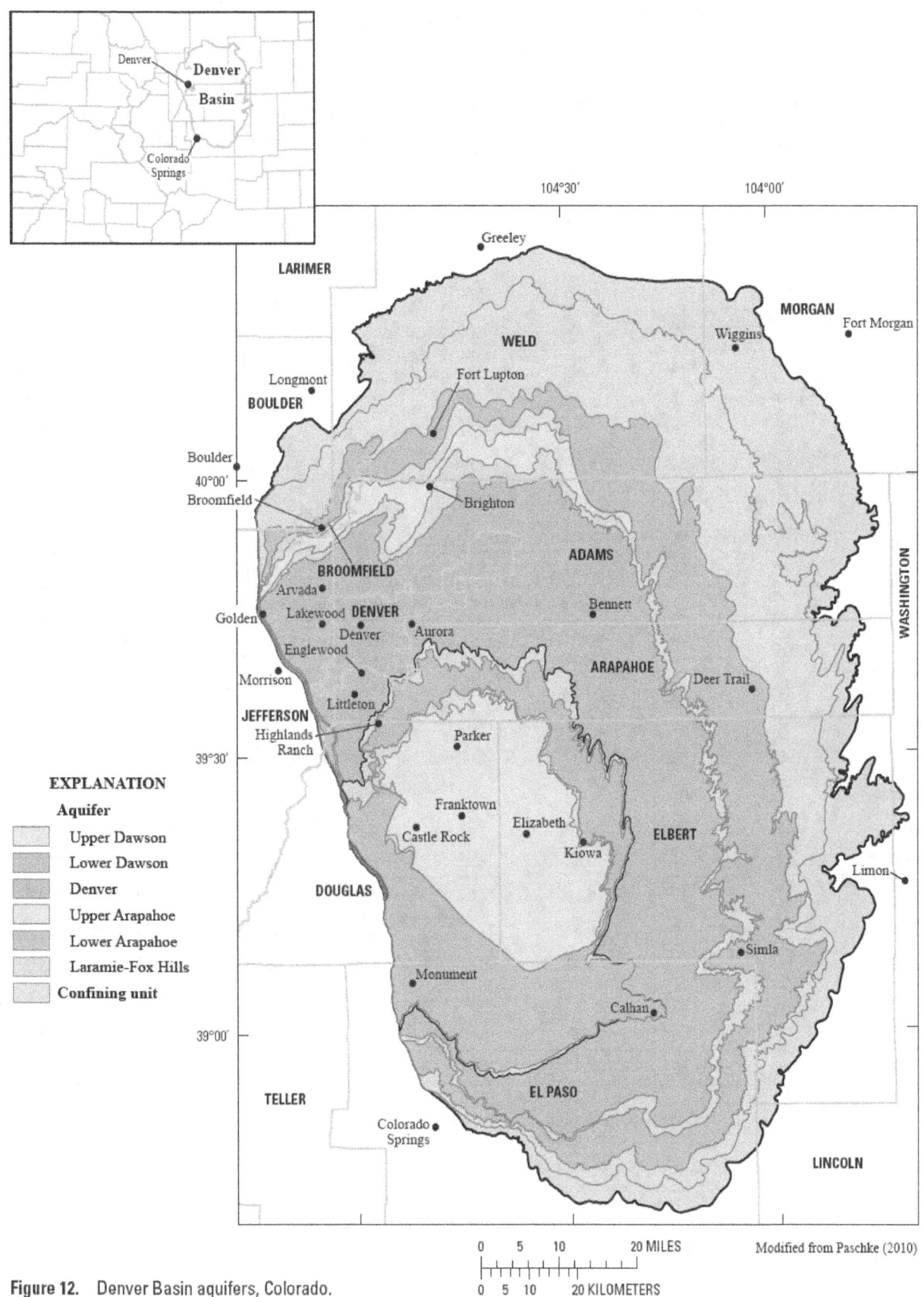

Figure 12. Denver Basin aquifers, Colorado.

Table 13.   Estimated water withdrawals from select aquifers, by county, Colorado, 2004.

[Data from Banta and others, 2010; Mgal/d, million gallons per day]

County (fig. 2)	Irrigation withdrawals (Mgal/d), for indicated aquifer							
	Alluvial	Upper Dawson	Lower Dawson	Denver	Upper Arapahoe	Lower Arapahoe	Laramie-Fox Hills	County total
Adams	18.20	0.00	0.00	2.52	3.38	0.87	0.66	25.63
Arapahoe	3.81	.00	0.11	1.37	1.00	2.76	.21	9.26
Boulder	.15	.00	.00	.00	.00	.00	.64	.79
Broomfield	.00	.00	.00	.00	.00	.00	.10	.10
Denver	3.04	.00	.00	.80	.15	.19	.08	4.26
Douglas	2.01	1.14	.55	.51	.00	.48	.04	4.73
Elbert	1.94	.75	.15	.48	.00	.53	.39	4.24
El Paso	6.08	.00	.33	.76	.00	1.45	.31	8.93
Jefferson	.40	.00	.00	1.69	.24	.29	.08	2.70
Morgan	15.75	.00	.00	.00	.00	.00	1.11	16.86
Weld	51.12	.00	.00	.03	.77	1.84	3.44	57.20
Total	102.50	1.89	1.14	8.16	5.54	8.41	7.06	134.70

County	Public-supply withdrawals (Mgal/d), for indicated aquifer							
	Alluvial	Upper Dawson	Lower Dawson	Denver	Upper Arapahoe	Lower Arapahoe	Laramie-Fox Hills	County total
Adams	2.27	0.00	0.00	22.48	33.10	39.12	23.76	120.73
Arapahoe	1.63	0.46	3.93	19.83	4.01	46.14	14.10	90.1
Boulder	.00	.00	.00	.00	.00	.00	12.89	12.89
Broomfield	.00	.00	.00	.00	.00	.00	2.82	2.82
Denver	.45	.00	.00	3.97	1.00	2.01	1.21	8.64
Douglas	.41	8.21	13.68	44.95	.00	95.29	10.87	173.41
Elbert	.23	3.19	6.38	6.61	.00	4.01	.40	20.82
El Paso	.36	.00	19.60	21.82	.00	68.21	15.30	125.29
Jefferson	.18	.00	.00	6.61	5.02	17.05	6.04	34.9
Morgan	.14	.00	.00	.00	.00	.00	.40	.54
Weld	1.72	.00	.00	.00	2.01	1.00	12.89	17.62
Total	7.39	11.86	43.59	126.27	45.14	272.83	100.68	607.76

Table 13. Estimated water withdrawals from select aquifers, by county, Colorado, 2004. —Continued

[Data from Banta and others, 2010; Mgal/d, million gallons per day]

County (fig. 2)	Commercial/industrial withdrawals (Mgal/d), for indicated aquifer							
	Alluvial	Upper Dawson	Lower Dawson	Denver	Upper Arapahoe	Lower Arapahoe	Laramie-Fox Hills	County total
Adams	0.78	0.00	0.00	0.35	0.39	0.73	0.23	2.48
Arapahoe	.28	.00	.09	.29	.17	.40	.18	1.41
Boulder	.00	.00	.00	.00	.00	.00	.27	.27
Broomfield	.00	.00	.00	.00	.00	.02	.07	.09
Denver	.40	.00	.00	.21	.07	.16	.02	.86
Douglas	.07	0.19	.45	.70	.00	.51	.06	1.98
Elbert	.03	.25	.16	.14	.00	.11	.06	.75
El Paso	.11	.00	.64	.58	.00	.40	.24	1.97
Jefferson	.35	.00	.00	.75	.13	.25	.12	1.60
Morgan	.15	.00	.00	.00	.00	.00	.02	.17
Weld	1.02	.00	.00	.00	.01	.08	.90	2.01
Total	3.19	0.44	1.34	3.02	0.77	2.66	2.17	13.59

County	Household (domestic) withdrawals (Mgal/d), for indicated aquifer							
	Alluvial	Upper Dawson	Lower Dawson	Denver	Upper Arapahoe	Lower Arapahoe	Laramie-Fox Hills	County total
Adams	0.00	0.00	0.00	0.01	0.01	0.03	0.00	0.05
Arapahoe	.00	.00	.00	.01	.00	.00	.00	.02
Boulder	.00	.00	.00	.00	.00	.00	.06	.06
Broomfield	.00	.00	.00	.00	.00	.00	.00	.00
Denver	.00	.00	.00	.00	.00	.00	.00	.00
Douglas	.00	.05	.07	.01	.00	.01	.01	.14
Elbert	.00	.07	.00	.00	.00	.00	.00	.08
El Paso	.00	.00	.23	.03	.00	.05	.01	.32
Jefferson	.00	.00	.00	.02	.01	.01	.00	.05
Morgan	.00	.00	.00	.00	.00	.00	.00	.00
Weld	.02	.00	.00	.00	.01	.01	.03	.07
Total	.02	0.12	0.31	0.08	0.03	0.11	0.11	0.79

Table 13.   Estimated water withdrawals from select aquifers, by county, Colorado, 2004.—Continued

[Data from Banta and others, 2010; Mgal/d, million gallons per day]

County (fig. 2)	Domestic/livestock withdrawals (Mgal/d), for indicated aquifer							
	Alluvial	Upper Dawson	Lower Dawson	Denver	Upper Arapahoe	Lower Arapahoe	Laramie-Fox Hills	County total
Adams	0.61	0.00	0.00	0.67	0.65	0.77	0.25	2.95
Arapahoe	.19	.02	0.30	.00	.10	.27	.13	1.01
Boulder	.01	.00	.00	.00	.00	.002	.64	.65
Broomfield	.00	.00	.00	.00	.01	.04	.03	.08
Denver	.04	.00	.00	.10	.01	.004	.00	.15
Douglas	.02	1.68	1.16	.68	.00	.16	.02	3.72
Elbert	.09	1.62	.57	.73	.00	.33	.20	3.54
El Paso	.35	.00	3.43	2.28	.00	1.10	.38	7.54
Jefferson	.18	.00	.00	1.09	.20	.17	.03	1.67
Lincoln	.00	.00	.00	.00	.00	.00	.002	.01
Morgan	.20	.00	.00	.00	.00	.00	.09	.29
Weld	.96	.00	.00	.00	.17	.25	1.20	2.58
Total	2.65	3.32	5.46	5.55	1.14	3.10	2.97	24.20
Aquifer totals	**115.77**	**17.64**	**51.84**	**143.08**	**52.62**	**287.11**	**112.99**	

estimate. Only one county, Mineral County, had an estimate nearly identical in both the SWSI baseline forecasted water demand and the USGS compilation. Differences for all the counties ranged from 0.1 to 299.28 percent with a median of 37.96 percent. Because the water-use categories of municipal and industrial were combined in the SWSI water-demand estimates, it is difficult to discern which water-use category had a difference between the SWSI forecast and the USGS compilation. However, differences between the SWSI water-demand estimates and USGS compilation estimates may be due to increased conservation efforts, which were not included in the water demand forecasts, as well as the differing methodology in deriving the forecasted and estimated values.

Ten counties had a 2005 thermoelectric water-use estimate reported in the SWSI forecast, whereas 13 counties were reported in the USGS compilation. A comparison of the withdrawal estimates between the SWSI forecast and the USGS compilation for those 10 counties showed that one county had a difference between −10 and 10 percent and four counties had a difference between −100 and 100 percent (table 14). Differences for the power generation water-use category ranged from −37.27 to 133.95 percent with a median of 7.11 percent.

Table 14. Comparison of 2005 Colorado Statewide Water Supply Initiative forecasted population and water demand and U.S. Geological Survey compilation estimates for population, municipal (public-supply) and industrial (combined), and thermoelectric power generation water use.

[SWSI, Colorado Statewide Water Supply Initiative; USGS, U.S. Geological Survey; Mgal/d, million gallons per day; --, not applicable]

County (fig. 2)	Population (thousands)			Municipal and industrial (Mgal/d)			Self-supplied power generation (Mgal/d)		
	SWSI	USGS	Percent difference	SWSI	USGS	Percent difference, relative to SWSI value	SWSI	USGS	Percent difference, relative to SWSI value
Adams	396.33	399.43	0.78	66.06	53.51	-19.00	8.54	9.25	8.31
Alamosa	16.04	15.28	-4.74	4.31	2.00	-53.60	.00	.00	--
Arapahoe	526.54	529.09	.48	103.04	75.69	-26.54	.00	.00	--
Archuleta	12.10	11.89	-1.74	2.57	.77	-70.04	.00	.00	--
Baca	4.23	4.07	-3.78	1.08	.75	-30.56	.00	.00	--
Bent	6.16	5.56	-9.74	1.12	1.13	.89	.00	.00	--
Boulder	288.65	280.44	-2.84	61.08	46.03	-24.64	2.61	5.82	122.99
Broomfield	43.94	43.48	-1.05	9.63	4.45	-53.79	.00	.00	--
Chaffee	17.42	16.97	-2.58	5.40	1.69	-68.70	.00	.00	--
Cheyenne	2.14	1.95	-8.88	.45	.44	-2.22	.00	.00	--
Clear Creek	9.70	9.20	-5.15	2.74	1.37	-50.00	.00	.00	--
Conejos	8.50	8.51	.12	3.61	.87	-75.90	.00	.00	--
Costilla	3.84	3.42	-10.94	.53	.43	-18.87	.00	.00	--
Crowley	5.76	5.40	-6.25	.82	.79	-3.66	.00	.00	--
Custer	4.06	3.86	-4.93	.92	.12	-86.96	.00	.00	--
Delta	30.83	29.95	-2.85	6.47	6.12	-5.41	.00	.00	--
Denver	574.32	557.92	-2.86	128.99	232.74	80.43	2.11	2.26	7.11
Dolores	1.97	1.83	-7.11	.40	.32	-20.00	.00	.00	--
Douglas	224.96	249.42	10.87	48.37	30.17	-37.63	.00	.00	--
Eagle	49.60	47.53	-4.17	14.19	9.45	-33.40	.00	.00	--
Elbert	23.81	22.79	-4.28	2.70	1.05	-61.11	.00	.00	--
El Paso	561.85	565.58	.66	109.89	116.66	6.16	--	2.54	--

Table 14. Comparison of 2005 Colorado Statewide Water Supply Initiative forecasted population and water demand and U.S. Geological Survey compilation estimates for population, municipal (public-supply) and industrial (combined), and thermoelectric power generation water use. —Continued

[SWSI, Colorado Statewide Water Supply Initiative; USGS, U.S. Geological Survey; Mgal/d, million gallons per day; --, not applicable]

County (fig. 2)	Population (thousands)			Municipal and industrial (Mgal/d)			Self-supplied power generation (Mgal/d)		
	SWSI	USGS	Percent difference	SWSI	USGS	Percent difference, relative to SWSI value	SWSI	USGS	Percent difference, relative to SWSI value
Fremont	48.81	47.77	-2.13	11.32	8.09	-28.53	--	15.48	--
Garfield	50.90	49.81	-2.14	11.45	15.12	32.05	0.00	0.00	--
Gilpin	4.94	4.93	-.20	1.02	.51	-50.00	.00	.00	--
Grand	14.26	13.21	-7.36	3.02	3.78	25.17	.00	.00	--
Gunnison	14.10	14.23	.92	2.65	3.50	32.08	.00	.00	--
Hinsdale	.82	.77	-6.10	.17	.51	200.00	.00	.00	--
Huerfano	8.46	7.77	-8.16	1.16	.85	-26.72	.00	.00	--
Jackson	1.63	1.45	-11.04	.44	.20	-54.55	.00	.00	--
Jefferson	543.60	526.80	-3.09	88.97	49.01	-44.91	--	.03	--
Kiowa	1.53	1.45	-7.19	.50	.14	-72.00	.00	.00	--
Kit Carson	8.13	7.64	-6.03	2.45	1.51	-38.37	--	.01	--
Lake	8.03	7.74	-3.61	1.70	1.27	-25.29	.00	.00	--
La Plata	48.26	47.45	-1.68	9.29	5.66	-39.07	4.60	.00	--
Larimer	270.44	271.93	.55	65.23	60.09	-7.88	.00	.00	--
Las Animas	16.63	15.45	-7.10	3.69	2.40	-34.96	.00	.00	--
Lincoln	6.12	5.62	-8.17	1.55	.81	-47.74	.00	.00	--
Logan	22.39	20.72	-7.46	4.03	2.54	-36.97	.00	.00	--
Mesa	129.39	129.87	.37	19.99	15.13	-24.31	--	43.85	--
Mineral	.91	.93	2.20	.27	.27	.00	.00	.00	--
Moffat	13.75	13.42	-2.40	2.61	1.60	-38.70	10.93	12.81	17.20
Montezuma	25.55	24.78	-3.01	5.52	2.64	-52.17	.00	.00	--
Montrose	38.12	37.48	-1.68	7.89	10.64	34.85	1.66	1.68	1.20

Table 14. Comparison of 2005 Colorado Statewide Water Supply Initiative forecasted population and water demand and U.S. Geological Survey compilation estimates for population, municipal (public-supply) and industrial (combined), and thermoelectric power generation water use.—Continued

[SWSI, Colorado Statewide Water Supply Initiative; USGS, U.S. Geological Survey; Mgal/d, million gallons per day; --, not applicable]

County (fig. 2)	Population (thousands)			Municipal and industrial (Mgal/d)			Self-supplied power generation (Mgal/d)		
	SWSI	USGS	Percent difference	SWSI	USGS	Percent difference, relative to SWSI value	SWSI	USGS	Percent difference, relative to SWSI value
Morgan	29.03	27.99	-3.58	9.89	7.07	-28.51	5.29	3.94	-25.52
Otero	19.62	19.50	-.61	4.77	5.07	6.29	.00	.00	--
Ouray	4.18	4.26	1.91	1.60	0.49	-69.38	0.00	0.00	--
Park	17.40	16.95	-2.59	3.45	.90	-73.91	.00	.00	--
Phillips	4.60	4.59	-.22	1.64	1.66	1.22	.00	.00	--
Pitkin	16.82	14.91	-11.36	11.47	4.38	-61.81	.00	.00	--
Prowers	14.29	13.89	-2.80	4.10	2.05	-50.00	.00	.00	--
Pueblo	153.99	151.32	-1.73	39.13	156.24	299.28	8.07	18.88	133.95
Rio Blanco	6.08	5.97	-1.81	1.78	3.55	99.44	.00	.00	--
Rio Grande	12.77	12.23	-4.23	5.18	1.40	-72.97	.00	.00	--
Routt	21.52	21.31	-.98	5.10	7.56	48.24	2.37	2.52	6.33
Saguache	6.56	7.03	7.16	2.18	.78	-64.22	.00	.00	--
San Juan	.58	.58	.00	.12	.24	100.00	.00	.00	--
San Miguel	7.77	7.21	-7.33	1.95	.75	-61.54	.00	.00	--
Sedgwick	2.78	2.53	-8.99	.87	.63	-27.59	.00	.00	--
Summit	28.25	24.89	-11.89	9.24	6.08	-34.20	.00	.00	--
Teller	23.11	21.92	-5.15	4.00	2.53	-36.75	.00	.00	--
Washington	4.90	4.63	-5.51	1.53	.69	-54.90	.00	.00	--
Weld	217.73	228.94	5.15	62.23	29.65	-52.35	6.60	4.14	-37.27
Yuma	10.02	9.79	-2.30	2.64	2.07	-21.59	.00	.00	--

Comparison of 1985 to 2005 Colorado Compilation Water Withdrawal Estimates

A generalized comparison of the published 1985 estimates to water withdrawal estimates 20 years later in 2005 can provide some indication of State water-use trends. An analysis of county-level trends with inclusion of intervening compilation years (1990, 1995, and 2000) would provide a more detailed picture of water-use/withdrawal trends in Colorado, but is beyond the scope of this report. Some differences exist in data collection and reporting methodologies between 1985 and 2005, including some optional categories in 2005, such as consumptive use (all categories), commercial water use, and hydroelectric power, and the separation of aquaculture from livestock and commercial categories. Total irrigation

estimates were compared between 1985 and 2005, as crop and golf course irrigation estimates were assumed to be totaled for 1985. All 1985 estimates were reported in Litke and Appel (1989).

Comparisons are provided for the following categories: irrigation (including irrigated acres), public supply (including population), self-supplied domestic (including population), self-supplied industrial, livestock, mining, and thermoelectric. Self-supplied commercial water use was estimated at 8.4 Mgal/d in 1985 but estimates were not compiled in 2005. Total withdrawals for the seven water-use categories compared between 1985 and 2005 did not differ greatly and indicated an increase of less than 1 percent (table 15). Most categories indicated an increase in water use in the 20 years from 1985 to 2005, including public supply, self-supplied domestic,

Table 15.   Comparison of Colorado total withdrawal estimates, by select category, 1985 and 2005.

[Data for 1985 estimates reported in Litke and Appel (1989); Mgal/d, million gallons per day; NA, not available]

Category	1985	2005	Percent increase or decrease, 1985–2005
Water use (Mgal/d)			
Total withdrawals	13,549.67	13,581.22	0.2
Irrigation	12,413.70	12,362.49	-.4
Irrigation—groundwater	2,128.28	2,357.82	10.8
Irrigation—surface water	10,285.42	10,004.67	-2.7
Public supply	737.08	864.17	17.2
Public supply groundwater	86.00	101.86	18.4
Public supply surface water	651.08	762.31	17.1
Self-supplied domestic	16.70	34.43	106.2
Self-supplied industrial	120.35	142.44	18.4
Livestock	60.74	33.06	-45.6
Mining	91.32	21.42	-76.5
Thermoelectric	109.78	123.21	12.2
Population (thousands)			
Served by public supply—groundwater	446.96	667.07	49.3
Served by public supply—surface water	2,562.51	3,689.50	44.0
Self-supplied domestic	221.73	298.61	34.7
Irrigated acres (thousands)			
Total irrigated acres	3,353.07	3,023.25	-9.8
Irrigated acres flood	2,678.57	1,875.24	-30.0
Irrigated acres sprinkler	674.50	1,147.57	70.1
Irrigated acres microirrigation	NA	3.16	NA

self-supplied industrial, and thermoelectric. These water-use categories can be directly linked to population increases and reflect the overall State population growth from 3.2 million in 1985 to 4.7 million in 2005 (U.S. Census Bureau, 2009). Table 15 lists the Colorado population served by public supply for both groundwater and surface water, and self-supplied domestic populations. These populations increased by 49.3, 44.0, and 34.7 percent respectively, from 1985 to 2005. Withdrawals for public supply increased 17.2 percent, whereas self-supplied domestic withdrawals increased 106.2 percent. As a consequence of increased population and the need for more manufactured and processed goods and electricity, water withdrawals for self-supplied industrial use increased 18.4 percent and thermoelectric generation increased 12.2 percent during the 20-year span.

Several water-use categories decreased between 1985 and 2005, including irrigation, livestock, and mining. Irrigation estimates decreased the least during these 20 years, less than 1 percent, from 12,413.70 Mgal/d in 1985 to 12,362.49 in 2005. However, when comparing the type of irrigated acres the differences are more pronounced. Overall, the estimates of total crop irrigated acres in Colorado decreased from 1985 to 2005 by almost 10 percent, from about 3,354 to 3,023 thousand acres, and the number of flood irrigated acres decreased by 30 percent. The number of acres for the more efficient sprinkler irrigation method increased substantially between 1985 and 2005, increasing by about 70 percent. Microirrigated acres were not reported in 1985, but totaled 3,160 acres in 2005. Withdrawals for livestock decreased from 60.74 Mgal/d in 1985 to 33.06 Mgal/d in 2005, a decrease of 45.6 percent. Mining withdrawals, decreased 69.9 Mgal/d or 76.5 percent in the intervening 20 years, reflecting the decrease in the number of coal and hard-rock mines from 150 in 1985 (Litke and Appel, 1989) to 20 in 2005.

Summary

Water is one of Colorado's most valued and vital resources, and a continuing supply of fresh water is important to the future health and economic welfare of the people and environment of Colorado. Comprehensive, current, and detailed water-use data will provide Colorado water managers and planners with information they need to quantify current stresses and estimate and plan for future water needs. The purpose of this report is to summarize the estimated amount of water withdrawn and used from Colorado's groundwater and surface-water resources, collected as part of the U.S. Geological Survey (USGS) National Water Use Information Program's data collection effort for 2005. This report is published in cooperation with the Colorado Water Conservation Board. Water withdrawals in Colorado are summarized for each of the following categories: irrigation (crop and golf course), public supply, self-supplied domestic, self-supplied industrial, livestock, mining, thermoelectric power generation, and instream

hydroelectric power generation. Water withdrawal and use estimates for each category are reported by water source and county and are summarized by Colorado river basins (four-digit hydrologic unit code (HUC)).

In 2005, an estimated 13,581.22 million gallons per day (Mgal/d) was withdrawn from groundwater and surface-water sources in Colorado for the seven water-use categories (excluding hydroelectric power generation). Withdrawals from surface water represented about 11,035 Mgal/d, or 81.3 percent of the total, whereas withdrawals from groundwater sources represented an estimated 2,546 Mgal/d, or 18.7 percent of the total. The counties with the largest total withdrawals (greater than 500 Mgal/d), excluding hydroelectric, were Mesa, Weld, Rio Grande, Montrose, Gunnison, and Saguache. Counties with the smallest total withdrawals (less than 5 Mgal/d) were Clear Creek, Gilpin, and San Juan. Four-digit HUCs with the greatest withdrawals were 1019 (South Platte River Basin), 1301 (Rio Grande Basin), and 1102 (Arkansas River Basin); the high withdrawal rates were driven by crop irrigation withdrawals.

Irrigation (crop and golf course) accounted for the largest withdrawals in Colorado (12,362.49 Mgal/d), which includes water used by crops as well as water lost through conveyances and return flows. Approximately 91 percent of the total water withdrawals in Colorado in 2005 was for irrigation. Eighty-one percent (10,004.67 Mgal/d) of irrigation water was supplied from surface-water sources. Irrigated crop land (including pasture) totaled 2,998,480 acres. A total estimated 12,321.85 Mgal/d of water was withdrawn for crop irrigation. Mesa, Weld, Rio Grande, Montrose, Saguache, and Gunnison Counties had the largest irrigation withdrawals (more than 500 Mgal/d), with Mesa, Weld, and Rio Grande Counties each using about 6 to 7 percent of the total irrigation withdrawals. Consumptive use is estimated to be 55.1 percent of the total withdrawals for irrigation, and the average consumptive-use rate for irrigated acres was about 2.54 acre-feet per irrigated acre. In 2005, Colorado had 243 turf golf courses across the State that had an estimated 2.27 acre-ft per irrigated course acre, and used 0.3 percent (40.64 Mgal/d) of the total irrigation water use.

In 2005, there were 844 community water systems (CWSs) in Colorado, including three tribal systems. The total quantity of water withdrawn for public-supply use in 2005 was estimated to be 864.17 Mgal/d, and the estimated number of people served in Colorado was 4.367 million or about 94 percent of the total population in the State. The majority of the drinking water for Coloradans came from a surface-water source (88.2 percent), and the counties with the largest surface-water withdrawals (greater than 50 Mgal/d) were Denver, El Paso, Pueblo, Arapahoe, and Larimer. The remaining 11.8 percent of public-supply water came from groundwater sources, and the counties with the greatest groundwater withdrawals were Douglas, El Paso, and Adams Counties.

In Colorado, all self-supplied domestic water use is from a groundwater source, and well withdrawals for 2005 totaled 34.43 Mgal/d, serving an estimated population of

298,610. Counties with the largest withdrawals (greater than 1 Mgal/d) were Jefferson, Weld, El Paso, Delta, Elbert, Park, and Garfield. The average estimated domestic per capita water use was 115 gallons per day (gal/d). Consumptive use for self-supplied domestic water was assumed to be 10 percent of withdrawals and was estimated as 3.44 Mgal/d.

In 2005, a total of 7,342 industries were located in Colorado, of which the principal employing industry groups in the State (in decreasing order of approximate number of employees) were communications equipment, newspapers, air/spacecraft manufacturers, prepackaged computer software, and commercial printers. Self-supplied industrial-water withdrawals in Colorado totaled an estimated 142.44 Mgal/d and ranged from little or no industrial water withdrawn in many counties to greater than 30 Mgal/d in Jefferson and Pueblo Counties. Surface water supplied 97.5 percent (138.83 Mgal/d) of the water to Colorado industries.

Water use for livestock constitutes less than 1 percent (33.06 Mgal/d) of the total water use in Colorado. Weld County had the greatest livestock withdrawals (7.12 Mgal/d groundwater and surface water combined). Other counties with greater than 2 Mgal/d livestock water use were Yuma, Morgan, and Logan. Groundwater supplied about 67 percent of the total livestock withdrawals (22.11 Mgal/d), whereas surface-water sources supplied about 10.95 Mgal/d. All water for livestock use was assumed to be consumptively used.

Total freshwater withdrawals for coal, hard-rock, and construction materials mining was estimated to be 5.20 Mgal/d from groundwater and 1.24 Mgal/d from surface water. Total water withdrawals for coal mining (both groundwater and fresh/saline surface water) were estimated to be 2.66 Mgal/d; hard-rock mines and sand/gravel quarries used about 0.01 and 4.17 Mgal/d, respectively, of groundwater resources only. For oil and gas wells, an estimated 14.59 Mgal/d of saline groundwater was withdrawn and reinjected. The counties with the largest amount of oil and gas production water use were Rio Blanco, Las Animas, and Moffat.

Total water withdrawn for 2005 thermoelectric power generation was 123.21 Mgal/d, of which surface-water sources accounted for 94.7 percent. Consumptive use was estimated to be 43.44 Mgal/d, with an average consumption rate for the 14 closed-loop plants of 84 percent of the withdrawn water. Counties with the greatest total withdrawals were Mesa, Pueblo, and Fremont. A total of about 38,174.40 gigawatt-hours of electricity were generated in 2005 by powerplants using water for cooling.

Total hydroelectric water use in 2005 was 5,253.6 Mgal/d, and produced 1,599.45 gigawatt-hours of electricity. Water used for the generation of hydroelectric power is considered an instream use and is nonconsumptive. In 2005, Colorado had 37 hydroelectric plants.

Groundwater withdrawals were estimated for the bedrock and overlying alluvial aquifers in the Denver Basin for irrigation, public supply, commercial/industrial, household-use-only, and domestic/livestock water-use categories. Withdrawals were estimated for input into the USGS Denver Basin

groundwater model using the equations in the Senate Bill 96-74 groundwater model. The bedrock aquifer units that make up the Denver Basin aquifer system are the Upper Dawson, Lower Dawson, Denver, Upper Arapahoe, Lower Arapahoe, and the Laramie-Fox Hills aquifers. A Quaternary-age alluvial aquifer overlies the Denver Basin aquifer system and was included in the withdrawal estimates. The greatest withdrawals were from public-supply wells and the smallest were from household-use-only wells. Douglas County had the greatest total withdrawals (183.98 Mgal/d), whereas Broomfield County had the smallest (3.09 Mgal/d). Of the seven Denver Basin aquifers, the Lower Arapahoe aquifer had the greatest total estimated withdrawals (287.11 Mgal/d), and Douglas County had the greatest public-supply withdrawal of any other county (95.29 Mgal/d) from this same aquifer. The Upper Dawson aquifer was the least used of the Denver Basin aquifers, based on an estimated total withdrawal of 17.64 Mgal/d.

As part of the Colorado Statewide Water Supply Initiative (SWSI), forecasts of future water demand were made based on information such as population, climate, and 2000 water-use information. These baseline water demand forecasts were made for municipal (public-supply), industrial, and select self-supplied (snow-making, power generation, and miscellaneous) water-use categories, and did not include the effects of future water conservation. Categories compared between estimates in the SWSI baseline-forecasted water demand and the USGS compilation were limited to county population and water use for public-supply/industrial and self-supplied thermoelectric power generation. Public-supply and industrial-water withdrawals are separate categories in the USGS compilation; however, these estimates were combined to compare to the SWSI municipal/industrial baseline-forecasted values.

Comparison of 2005 population estimates between the SWSI forecast and the USGS 2005 compilation showed that 40 of the 64 counties had a difference between −5 and 5 percent, and 59 of the counties (92 percent) had a difference between −10 and 10 percent. For all 64 counties, the population difference ranged from −11.89 to 10.87 percent with a median percent difference of −2.85. For the combined municipal and industrial categories, differences for all the counties ranged from −86.96 to 299.28 percent with a median of 31.98 percent. Of the 64 Colorado counties, 49 (77 percent) had a public-supply/industrial USGS withdrawal estimate that was lower than the SWSI water-demand estimate. Because the water-use categories of municipal and industrial were combined in the SWSI water demand estimates, it is difficult to discern which water-use category has a difference between the SWSI forecast and the USGS compilation. However, differences between the SWSI forecasted water demand and USGS compilation estimates may be due to increased conservation efforts, which were not included in the water-demand forecasts, and the differences in methodology in deriving the forecasted and estimated values. Ten counties had a 2005 thermoelectric power generation water-use estimate reported in the SWSI forecast; in the USGS compilation, 13 counties reported. Differences for the power generation water-use category ranged from –37.27 to 133.95 percent with a median of 7.11 percent.

A generalized comparison of the published 1985 estimates to water-use estimates 20 years later in 2005 can provide some indication of State water-use trends. An analysis of county-level trends with inclusion of intervening compilation years (1990, 1995, and 2000) would provide a more detailed picture of water-use/withdrawal trends in Colorado, but is beyond the scope of this report. Estimates of total water use were compared for irrigation (including irrigated acres), public supply (including population), self-supplied domestic (including population), self-supplied industrial, livestock, mining, and thermoelectric. Commercial water use was estimated in 1985 but was not compiled in 2005, and the irrigation estimates for 1985 are assumed to include golf course irrigation data. Total withdrawals for the seven categories compiled in 1985 and 2005 did not differ greatly and indicated an increase of less than 1 percent. A number of water-use categories indicated an increase in water withdrawals in the 20 years from 1985 to 2005; these included public supply, self-supplied domestic, self-supplied industrial, and thermoelectric. These water-use categories can be directly linked to population increases and reflect the overall State population growth from 3.2 million in 1985 to 4.7 million in 2005. Withdrawals for public supply increased 17.2 percent, whereas self-supplied domestic withdrawals increased 106.2 percent. As a consequence of increased population and the need for more manufactured and processed goods and electricity, water withdrawals for self-supplied industrial increased 18.4 percent and thermoelectric generation increased 12.2 percent between 1985 and 2005. A number of water-use categories decreased between 1985 and 2005, including irrigation, livestock, and mining. Irrigation estimates decreased the least during these 20 years, less than 1 percent, from 12,413.70 to 12,362.49 Mgal/d; however, irrigated acres decreased by approximately 10 percent (3,354 to 3,023 thousand acres). Withdrawals for livestock have decreased from 60.74 in 1985 to 33.06 Mgal/d in 2005, a decrease of 45.6 percent. Mining withdrawals, comparing 1985 to 2005 estimates, decreased 69.9 Mgal/d or 76.5 percent in the intervening 20 years, reflecting the decrease in the number of coal and hard-rock mines from 150 in 1985 to 20 in 2005.

Acknowledgments

The authors would like to thank Lori Gerzina of the Colorado Department of Public Health and Environment for sponsoring and distributing the public-supply water-use survey, and all the community water system managers and superintendents for their time and attention in completing the surveys. The authors also thank Joe McCleary, past President of the Rocky Mountain Golf Course Superintendents Association, for his assistance in sponsoring, designing, and distributing the Web-based golf course irrigation survey to the association members. The authors also thank all the association members who completed the survey for their time and attention as they provided valuable information on Colorado golf course irrigation and maintenance. Finally, the authors would like to thank Doug Stenzel of the Division of Water Resources for access to the 2005 water database (HydroBase), the Bureau of Reclamation, and powerplant personnel, coal and mineral mining personnel, water commissioners, and individual water users throughout the State for sharing water data and for their patience as the authors became familiar with the many ways water is used in Colorado.

References Cited

Banta, E.R., Paschke, S.S., and Litke, D.W., 2010, Groundwater flow simulations of the Denver Basin aquifer system, Colorado, chap. C of Pascke, S.S., ed. Groundwater availability of the Denver Basin Aquifer System, Colorado: U.S. Geological Survey Professional Paper 1770.

Blaney, H.F., Rich, L.R., and Criddle, W.D., and others, 1952, Consumptive use of water: Transactions of the American Society of Civil Engineers, no. 117, p. 948–967.

Cappa, J.A., Young, Genevieve, Keller, J.W., Carroll, C.J., and Widmann, Beth, 2006, Colorado mineral and energy industry activities, 2005: Colorado Geological Survey Information Series 73, accessed June 5, 2008, at *http://geosurvey.state.co.us/programs&projects/Mineral&EnergyResouces/Minerals/MineralResources.*

Colorado Department of Local Affairs, 2006, Section VI, Taxable real and personal property, agriculture: Colorado Department of Local Affairs, Division of Property Taxation, accessed February 10, 2006, at *http://www.dola.state.co.us/dpt/publications/annual_report_index.htm.*

Colorado Division of Reclamation Mining and Safety, 2008, DRMS reports: Colorado Division of Reclamation Mining and Safety, accessed June 12, 2008, at *http://mining.state.co.us/DMG%20Reports.htm.*

Colorado Division of Water Resources, 1998, Denver Basin and South Platte River basin technical study, final report: Senate Bill 96-074, variously paged.

Colorado Oil and Gas Conservation Commission, 2007, Colorado oil and gas information system, accessed June 29, 2007, at *http://oil-gas.state.co.us/Database/Production/.*

Colorado State University Extension Service, 2006, Irrigation scheduling—The water balance approach, accessed March 10, 2006, at *http://www.ext.colostate.edu/pubs/crops/04707.html.*

Colorado Water Conservation Board, 2004, Colorado Statewide Water Supply Initiative, SWSI Water Demand Forecast: Carbondale, Ill., Technical Memorandum 3.2, August 6, 2004, 131 p.

Colorado Water Conservation Board and Colorado Division of Water Resources, 2006, Colorado's decision support systems, 2006, Colorado Division of Water Resources, accessed March 20, 2006, at *http://cdss.state.co.us/docs/cdssBasins.aspx?category=2&basin=5.*

Hutson, S.S., Barber, N.L., Kenny, J.F., Linsey, K.S., Lumia, D.S., and Maupin, M.A., 2004, Estimated use of water in the United States in 2000: U.S. Geological Survey Circular 1268, 46 p.

Ivahnenko, Tamara, 2009, Estimated Colorado golf course irrigation water use: U.S. Geological Survey Open-File Report 2008–1267, 34 p.

Litke, D.W., and Appel, C.L., 1989, Estimated use of water in Colorado, 1985: U.S. Geological Survey Water-Resources Investigations Report 88–4101, 157 p.

Lovelace, J.K., 2009a, Method for estimating water withdrawals for livestock in the United States, 2005: U.S. Geological Survey Scientific Investigations Report 2009–5041, 7 p.

Lovelace, J.K., 2009b, Methods for estimating water withdrawals for mining in the United States, 2005: U.S. Geological Survey Scientific Investigations Report 2009–5053, 7 p.

MacKichan, K.A., 1951, Estimated use of water in the United States, 1950: U.S. Geological Survey Circular 115, 13 p.

MacKichan, K.A., 1957, Estimated use of water in the United States, 1955: U.S. Geological Survey Circular 389, 18 p.

MacKichan, K.A., and Kammerer, J.C., 1961, Estimated use of water in the United States, 1960: U.S. Geological Survey Circular 456, 44 p.

Manufacturers' News, Inc., 2005, Colorado manufacturers database: Evanston, Ill., Manufacturers' News, Inc., CD-ROM.

Murray, C.R., 1968, Estimated use of water in the United States, 1965: U.S. Geological Survey Circular 556, 53 p.

Murray, C.R., and Reeves, E.B., 1972, Estimated use of water in the United States in 1970: U.S. Geological Survey Circular 676, 37 p.

Murray, C.R., and Reeves, E.B., 1977, Estimated use of water in the United States in 1975: U.S. Geological Survey Circular 765, 39 p.

National Priorities Project Database, 2001, Energy statistics—renewable hydroelectric production; StateMaster.com, accessed June 12, 2008, at *http://www.statemaster.com/graph/ene_ren_hyd_pro-energy-renewable-hydroelectric-production.*

Paschke, S.S., ed., 2010, Groundwater availability of the Denver Basin aquifer system, Colorado: U.S. Geological Survey Professional Paper 1770, 302 p.

Solley, W.B., Chase, E.B., and Mann,W.B., IV, 1983, Estimated use of water in the United States in 1980: U.S. Geological Survey Circular 1001, 56 p.

Solley, W.B., Charles, F.M., and Pierce, R.R., 1988, Estimated use of water in the United States in 1980: U.S. Geological Survey Circular 1004, 82 p.

Solley, W.B., Pierce, R.R., and Perlman, H.A., 1993, Estimated use of water in the United States in 1990: U.S. Geological Survey Circular 1081, 76 p.

Solley, W.B., Pierce, R.R., and Perlman, H.A., 1998, Estimated use of water in the United States in 1995: U.S. Geological Survey Circular 1200, 71 p.

U.S. Census Bureau, 2006, Annual estimates of the population of counties of Colorado: April 1, 2000, to July 1, 2005: U.S. Census Bureau Population Estimates, CO-EST2005-01-08.

U.S. Census Bureau, 2009, Colorado quickfacts: U.S. Census Bureau State and County Quickfacts, accessed May 6, 2009, at *http://quickfacts.census.gov/qfd/states/08000lk.html.*

U.S. Department of Agriculture, 2002, Census of agriculture, United States summary and State data, Geographic Area Series AC-02-A-51, June 2004, part 51, v. 1, 633 p.

U.S. Department of Agriculture, 2006, National agricultural statistics service, State/county irrigated land, accessed March 10, 2006, at *http://www.nass.usda.gov/ind.*

U.S. Department of Energy, 2006, Energy Information Administration, Forms EIA-906, EIA-920, EIA-767: U.S. Department of Energy, accessed February 6, 2006 at *http://www.eia.doe.gov/oss/forms.html.*

U.S. Geological Survey, 2007, National land cover database (NLCD 2001) Multi-zone download site, accessed May 11, 2007, at *http://www.mrlc.gov/nlcd_multizone_map.php.*

U.S. Geological Survey, 2009, Ground water atlas of the United States: Arizona, Colorado, New Mexico and Utah, HA-730C, accessed December 14, 2009, at *http://pubs.usgs.gov/ha/ha730/ch_c/C-text6.html.*

U.S. Environmental Protection Agency, 2004, Guidelines for water reuse: U.S. Environmental Protection Agency EPA/625/R-04/108, September 2004, accessed January 8, 2010 at *http://www.epa.gov/nrmrl/pubs/625r04108/625r04108.pdf.*

U.S. Environmental Protection Agency, 2006, Safe drinking water information system: U.S. Environmental Protection Agency database, accessed January 10, 2006, at *http://www.epa.gov/safewater/database.html.*

U.S. Environmental Protection Agency, 2009, Basic information, Safe Drinking Water Act of 1974: U.S. Environmental Protection Agency, accessed January 5, 2009, at *http://www.epa.gov/safewater/sdwa/basicinformation.html.*

Glossary

Aquifer   A geological formation, group of formations, or part of a formation that contains sufficient saturated material to yield significant quantities of water to wells and springs.

Agricultural water use   Includes water used for irrigation and nonirrigation purposes. Irrigation water use includes the artificial application of water on lands to assist in the growing of crops and pasture, or to maintain vegetative growth in recreational lands, parks, and golf courses. Nonirrigation agricultural water use includes water used for livestock, which includes water for stock watering, feed-lots, dairy operations, fish farming, and other farm needs.

Commercial water use   Water use for motels, hotels, restaurants, office buildings, commercial facilities, and civilian and military institutions. The water can be obtained from a public supply or can be self supplied.

Consumptive use   That part of water withdrawn that is evaporated, transpired, incorporated into products or crops, consumed by humans or livestock, or otherwise removed from the immediate water environment. Consumptive use is sometimes called water consumed. Additionally, any water withdrawn in the basin and transferred out of the basin for use is considered 100 percent consumptively used.

Cooling water   Water used for cooling purposes, such as in condensers.

Conveyance loss   Water that is lost in transit from a pipe, canal, conduit, or ditch by leakage or evaporation. Generally, the water is not available for further use; however, leakage from an irrigation ditch, for example, may percolate to a groundwater source and/or return to a surface-water source and be available for further use.

Domestic water use   Water for normal household purposes such as drinking, food preparation, bathing, washing clothes and dishes, flushing toilets, and watering lawns and gardens. The water can be obtained from a public supply or can be self-supplied.

Flood irrigation   Irrigation systems that spread water on the land surface with a system of lateral supply ditches or conduits. These include open field ditch systems, semiclosed conveyance systems, subsurface conduit systems, and continuous flood systems.

Hydroelectric power water use   The use of water in the generation of electricity at plants where the turbine generators are driven by falling water. Hydroelectric power water use is considered an instream use of water, and generally is a nonconsumptive use of water.

Industrial water use   Water used for industrial purposes such as fabricating, processing, washing, and cooling, and includes water used for such industries as steel, chemical and allied products, paper and allied products, mining, and petroleum refining. The water can be obtained from a public supply or can be self-supplied.

Instream use   Water used within the stream channel for such purposes as hydroelectric power generation, navigation, water-quality improvement, fish and wildlife propagation, and recreation. Sometimes called non-withdrawal use or in-channel use.

Microirrigation   An irrigation system that wets only a discrete portion of the soil surface in the vicinity of the plant by means of applicators (orifices, emitters, porous tubing, perforated pipe, and so forth) operated under low pressure. The applicators can be placed on or below the surface of the ground or can be suspended from supports.

Public supply   Water withdrawn by public and private water suppliers and delivered to users. Public suppliers provide water for a variety of uses, such as domestic, commercial, industrial, thermoelectric power (domestic and cooling purposes), and public-water use. Also see domestic water use, commercial water use, industrial water use, public-water use, and other water use.

Public supply deliveries   The amount of water delivered from a public supplier to users for domestic, commercial, industrial, thermo-electric-power, or public-use purposes.

Public-water use   Water supplied from a public-water supply and used for such purposes as firefighting, street washing, municipal parks, and swimming pools. Public-water use also includes system water losses (water lost to leakage). Also referred to as water-utility use.

Return flow   Water that reaches a groundwater or surface-water source after release from the point of use and thus becomes available for further use.

Saline water   Water that has greater than 1,000 parts per million dissolved salts.

Self-supplied water   Water withdrawn from a groundwater or surface-water source by a user and not obtained from a public supply.

Sprinkler irrigation   A pressurized irrigation system where water is distributed through pipes to the field and applied through a variety of sprinkler heads or drop tubes and emitters. Pressure is used to spread water droplets above the crop canopy to simulate rainfall. These systems include portable and traveling gun systems, solid or permanent fixture systems, center pivot systems, and periodic moving systems.

Thermoelectric power   Electrical power generated by using fossil-fuel (coal, oil, or natural gas) or geothermal energy.

Thermoelectric-power water use   Water used in the process of the generation of thermoelectric power. The water can be obtained from a public supply or be self-supplied. Water used for thermoelectric power generation purposes is considered an offstream use of water, and can supply either a once-through or closed-loop facility. A once-through plant uses withdrawn water for cooling and the water is then returned to the hydrologic system, and is considered a nonconsumptive use. Closed-loop plants recirculate withdrawn water until complete consumption with no return flows.

Water transfer   Artificial conveyance of water from one area to another. This transfer may be referred to as an import or export of water from one basin or county to or from another.

Withdrawal   Water removed from the ground or diverted from a surface-water source for use.

Appendix

Appendix tables 1–1 through 1–9 list water withdrawals by four-digit hydrologic unit codes (HUCs) for the categories of irrigation (crop and golf course), public supply, self-supplied domestic, self-supplied industrial, mining, livestock, thermoelectric, and hydroelectric power generation. HUCs are shown in figure 1. Water withdrawal information for the four-digit HUCs was calculated by converting the county water-use estimates through various manual and computer (geographic information system) accounting methods.

Table 1-1.   Water withdrawals for crop irrigation in Colorado by four-digit hydrologic unit code, 2005.

[Mgal/d, million gallons per day]

Hydrologic unit code (fig. 1)	Irrigated acres (thousands)	Groundwater (Mgal/d)	Surface water (Mgal/d)	Consumptive use (Mgal/d)
1018	191.33	6.58	451.91	286.76
1019	464.45	320.03	1,674.20	1,396.19
1025	578.47	860.14	151.11	940.06
1026	46.26	72.52	.23	62.51
1102	400.86	97.10	1,493.15	1,043.14
1103	7.88	9.27	13.49	15.65
1104	109.08	145.45	83.25	182.48
1301	493.77	791.04	1,175.05	1,185.26
1302	11.02	10.36	31.59	26.33
1401	201.28	.97	1,700.77	388.47
1402	200.60	20.78	1,769.87	574.96
1403	32.87	2.08	168.51	87.71
1404	.06	.00	.41	.17
1405	117.32	9.56	535.91	256.60
1406	.03	.00	.20	.12
1408	143.19	4.19	722.12	336.81
Total	2,998.48	2,350.07	9,971.78	6,783.49

Table 1-2. Water withdrawals for golf course irrigation in Colorado by four-digit hydrologic unit code, 2005.

[Mgal/d, million gallons per day]

Hydrologic unit code (fig. 1)	Irrigated acres (thousands)	Groundwater (Mgal/d)	Surface water (Mgal/d)	Reclaimed wastewater (Mgal/d)
1018	0.00	0.00	0.00	0.00
1019	13.51	5.43	16.44	3.70
1025	.26	.47	.12	.00
1026	.05	.11	.00	.00
1102	4.29	1.25	2.93	1.69
1103	.00	.00	.00	.00
1104	.00	.00	.00	.00
1301	.27	.00	.34	.00
1302	.00	.00	.00	.00
1401	4.23	.05	7.95	.00
1402	.84	.00	2.26	.00
1403	.08	.00	.08	.00
1404	.00	.00	.00	.00
1405	.66	.01	1.95	.00
1406	.00	.00	.00	.00
1408	.63	.42	.86	.10
Total	24.80	7.72	32.92	5.49

Table 1-3.   Water withdrawals for public-supply and domestic deliveries in Colorado by four-digit hydrologic unit code, 2005.

[Mgal/d, million gallons per day; gal/d, gallons per day]

Hydrologic unit code (fig. 1)	Population served (thousands)		Withdrawals (Mgal/d)		Domestic water deliveries (Mgal/d)	Per capita domestic use (gal/d)
	Groundwater	Surface water	Groundwater	Surface water		
1018	0.42	0.38	0.08	0.10	0.48	600
1019	492.94	3,099.25	64.03	595.53	332.57	93
1025	14.03	.00	3.98	.00	2.94	210
1026	1.04	.00	.33	.00	.34	326
1102	45.17	225.97	9.99	96.74	132.36	488
1103	.00	.00	.00	.00	.00	0
1104	2.89	.00	.75	.00	.27	93
1301	29.45	.86	5.60	.14	4.58	151
1302	.05	.00	.01	.00	.00	0
1401	67.11	230.08	13.51	45.09	29.84	100
1402	10.00	50.88	1.86	13.90	12.29	202
1403	.83	29.49	.09	3.34	1.34	44
1404	.00	.00	.00	.00	.00	0
1405	2.59	11.60	.66	2.16	5.30	373
1406	.00	.00	.00	.00	.00	0
1408	10.55	41.17	.97	5.31	7.13	138
Total	677.07	3,689.50	101.86	762.31	529.51	121[1]

[1] Average per capita.

Table 1-4.   Water withdrawals for self-supplied domestic use in Colorado by four-digit hydrologic unit code, 2005.

[Mgal/d, million gallons per day]

Hydrologic unit code (fig. 1)	Self-supplied population (thousands)	Groundwater (Mgal/d)
1018	0.67	0.12
1019	179.95	16.19
1025	4.89	1.15
1026	.53	.15
1102	47.12	7.01
1103	.15	.02
1104	1.21	.11
1301	17.04	2.72
1302	.01	.00
1401	13.94	1.81
1402	11.94	2.40
1403	1.86	.19
1404	.04	.00
1405	9.23	1.53
1406	.00	.00
1408	10.03	1.03
Total	298.61	34.43

Table 1-5.   Water withdrawals for self-supplied industrial use in Colorado by four-digit hydrologic unit code, 2005.

[Mgal/d, million gallons per day]

Hydrologic unit code (fig. 1)	Groundwater (Mgal/d)	Surface water (Mgal/d)
1018	0.00	0.02
1019	3.61	53.61
1025	.00	.00
1026	.00	.02
1102	.00	73.79
1103	.00	.00
1104	.00	.00
1301	.00	.00
1302	.00	.00
1401	.00	2.71
1402	.00	2.49
1403	.00	.18
1404	.00	.00
1405	.00	5.34
1406	.00	.00
1408	.00	.67
Total	3.61	138.83

Table 1-6.   Water withdrawals for livestock in Colorado by four-digit hydrologic unit code, 2005.

[Mgal/d, million gallons per day]

Hydrologic unit code (fig. 1)	Groundwater (Mgal/d)	Surface water (Mgal/d)
1018	0.03	0.36
1019	11.31	2.95
1025	5.71	1.08
1026	.22	.05
1102	3.22	2.73
1103	.04	.03
1104	.05	.12
1301	.36	.50
1302	.01	.01
1401	.22	.65
1402	.33	.83
1403	.14	.41
1404	.03	.04
1405	.29	.68
1406	.00	.00
1408	.13	.52
Total	22.11	10.95

Table 1-7.   Water withdrawals for mining in Colorado by four-digit hydrologic unit code, 2005.

[Mgal/d, million gallons per day]

Hydrologic unit code (fig. 1)	Groundwater (Mgal/d)	Saline groundwater (Mgal/d)	Surface water (Mgal/d)	Saline surface water (Mgal/d)
1018	0.04	0.15	0.00	0.00
1019	1.19	1.66	.00	.00
1025	.35	.38	.00	.00
1026	.01	.19	.00	.00
1102	1.18	1.62	.00	.00
1103	.00	.02	.00	.00
1104	.05	.29	.00	.00
1301	.20	.00	.00	.00
1302	.00	.00	.00	.00
1401	.39	.00	.00	.00
1402	.84	.00	.23	.00
1403	.09	.00	.43	.00
1404	.00	.00	.00	.00
1405	.72	9.95	.58	.39
1406	.00	.00	.00	.00
1408	.15	.33	.00	.00
Total	5.20	14.59	1.24	0.39

Table 1-8.   Water withdrawals for thermoelectric power generation in Colorado by four-digit hydrologic unit code, 2005.

[Mgal/d, million gallons per day; GWh, gigawatt-hours]

Hydrologic unit code (fig. 1)	Groundwater (Mgal/d)	Surface water (Mgal/d)	Consumptive use (Mgal/d)	Power generated (GWh)
1018	0.00	0.00	0.00	0.00
1019	3.59	21.49	18.16	13,807.74
1025	.01	.00	.00	1.82
1026	.00	.00	.00	.00
1102	2.54	34.36	8.53	6,349.48
1103	.00	.00	.00	.00
1104	.00	.00	.00	.00
1301	.00	.00	.00	.00
1302	.00	.00	.00	.00
1401	.00	43.85	.00	3,972.10
1402	.00	.00	.00	.00
1403	.00	1.68	1.42	736.96
1404	.00	.00	.00	.00
1405	.00	15.33	15.32	13,262.55
1406	.00	.00	.00	.00
1408	.00	.00	.00	43.75
Total	6.50	116.71	43.44	38,174.40

Table 1-9.   Instream water use for hydroelectric power generation in Colorado by four-digit hydrologic unit code, 2005.

[Mgal/d, million gallons per day; GWh, gigawatt-hours]

Hydrologic unit code (fig. 1)	Surface water (Mgal/d)	Power generated (GWh)
1018	0.00	0.00
1019	962.92	457.64
1025	.00	.00
1026	.00	.00
1102	163.28	84.57
1103	.00	.00
1104	.00	.00
1301	.00	.00
1302	.00	.00
1401	1,265.16	147.55
1402	2,064.37	686.94
1403	193.00	7.74
1404	.00	.00
1405	53.87	11.61
1406	.00	.00
1408	551.00	203.40
Total	5,253.60	1,599.45

www.ingramcontent.com/pod-product-compliance
Lightning Source LLC
Chambersburg PA
CBHW080437290526
45791CB00008BA/2531